Sex and Intimacy in Later Life

Series Editors: **Paul Simpson**, University of Manchester, **Paul Reynolds**, International Network for Sexual Ethics and Politics and The Open University and **Trish Hafford-Letchfield**, University of Strathclyde

Older people are commonly characterised as non-sexual, or their sexuality is considered a superficial concern in comparison to health, public services and pensions. This is despite evidence of an increase in sexual engagement amongst older people. Little academic attention has been given to this subject, or to the impact that this may have, such as increased rates of STI transmission or implications of healthy sex lives for care institutions.

This new, internationally-focused series will build on, extend and deepen knowledge of sexual practice amongst older people. Pulling together work by established and emerging scholars across a range of disciplines, it will cover the experiential, empirical and theoretical landscapes of sex and ageing.

Also available

Desexualisation in Later Life
The Limits of Sex and Intimacy
Edited by **Paul Simpson**, **Paul Reynolds** and **Trish Hafford-Letchfield**

Sex and Diversity in Later Life
Critical Perspectives
Edited by **Trish Hafford-Letchfield**, **Paul Simpson** and **Paul Reynolds**

Forthcoming in the series

Resexualising Later Life
Performances of Older Sexual and Intimate Citizenship
Edited by **Paul Reynolds**, **Trish Hafford-Letchfield** and **Paul Simpson**

Find out more at
policy.bristoluniversitypress.co.uk/
sex-and-intimacy-in-later-life

Sex and Intimacy in Later Life

Series Editors: **Paul Simpson**, University of Manchester, **Paul Reynolds**, International Network for Sexual Ethics and Politics and The Open University and **Trish Hafford-Letchfield**, University of Strathclyde

Find out more at
policy.bristoluniversitypress.co.uk/
sex-and-intimacy-in-later-life

HIV, SEX AND SEXUALITY IN LATER LIFE

Edited by
Mark Henrickson, Casey Charles, Shiv Ganesh, Sulaimon
Giwa, Kan Diana Kwok and Tetyana Semigina

With a foreword by
OmiSoore H. Dryden

First published in Great Britain in 2023 by

Policy Press, an imprint of
Bristol University Press
University of Bristol
1–9 Old Park Hill
Bristol
BS2 8BB
UK
t: +44 (0)117 374 6645
e: bup-info@bristol.ac.uk

Details of international sales and distribution partners are available at
policy.bristoluniversitypress.co.uk

British Library Cataloguing in Publication Data
A catalogue record for this book is available from the British Library

ISBN 978-1-4473-6197-8 hardcover
ISBN 978-1-4473-6198-5 ePub
ISBN 978-1-4473-6199-2 ePdf

Cover design: Robin Hawes
Front cover image: Getty/4FR
Bristol University Press and Policy Press use environmentally responsible
print partners.
Printed and bound in Great Britain by CPI Group (UK) Ltd, Croydon, CR0 4YY

FSC
www.fsc.org
MIX
Paper | Supporting
responsible forestry
FSC® C013604

Contents

Notes on contributors

Casey Charles lives in Palm Springs, California, and Missoula, Montana, where he has taught queer studies, law in literature, and Shakespeare. He has published non-fiction, a collection of essays, two novels and a poetry collection. His writing draws on his experience as an activist and attorney. *Undetectable*, his forthcoming memoir from Running Wild Press, puts the story of an HIV-positive gay man in America next to the long-term survival narratives of positive women and men from India and Kenya. Visit his website at www.caseycharles.com.

Cesare Di Feliciantonio is Senior Lecturer in Human Geography at Manchester Metropolitan University, UK. For the period 2018–20 he was the recipient of a Marie Skłodowska-Curie Actions Individual Fellowship (at the University of Leicester, UK). He is a co-editor of *ACME: An International Journal for Critical Geographies*. His work has been published in, among others: *Antipode*; *Cities*; *Gender, Place & Culture*; *Geoforum*; *International Journal of Urban and Regional Research*; *Social & Cultural Geography*; and *Urban Geography*.

Vanessa Fargnoli is a sociologist specialising in health, HIV/AIDS and qualitative methods. Her PhD thesis (2019) was titled *Living with HIV: An Invisible Condition. Trajectories of HIV-Infected Women in the French-Speaking Part of Switzerland* and published as a book in 2021 under the title of *INvihSIBLES. Trajectoires de femmes séropositives* (Lausanne, Editions Antipodes). She is also author of the book *Viol(s) comme arme de guerre* (Paris, L'Harmattan, 2012) based on her Master's thesis in health anthropology.

Shiv Ganesh is Professor of Communication Studies in the Moody College of Communication at The University of Texas at Austin. He studies communication and collective organising in the context of globalisation and digital technologies. He has done fieldwork in a number of countries, including Aotearoa New Zealand, India, Sweden and the United States. Current projects include a study of advocacy and voice among Indigenous people displaced by the creation of environmental reserves in India, a large-scale survey of digital interaction and engagement dynamics among global networks of activists, and an examination of transparency issues in environmentalism.

Sulaimon Giwa is Associate Professor and Associate Dean of Social Work at Memorial University. He has over a decade of experience in research, policy and direct practice at the community and federal levels, in health promotions, community and organisational practice in diverse communities, forensic social work and corrections and policing. His interdisciplinary and applied research programme and professional activities centralise LGBTQ2S+ experiences, intersectional stigmas and health related quality of life, and understanding of structural racism in the criminal justice system, from a critical race transformative lens.

Mark Henrickson is Professor of Social Work at Massey University, Auckland, Aotearoa New Zealand. He worked for many years in HIV-related healthcare. He has published extensively on gender and sexually diverse populations, and led the AfricaNZ Health study on HIV and Black African new settlers in Aotearoa New Zealand. Recent publications include the edited book *Getting to Zero: Global Social Work Responds to HIV* (available free from the UNAIDS website) and the monograph *The Origins of Social Care and Social Work* (2022). His current research explores the ethics of intimacy and sexuality in residential aged care. His PhD is from UCLA.

Kanamik Kani Khan is Lecturer in Social Work at the University of Essex and a registered social worker in England. He teaches both BA and MA modules, and supervises dissertations and students on placements. He was previously a lecturer at the Eastern Institute of Technology, Aotearoa New Zealand. He holds a PhD in social work from Massey University, Aotearoa New Zealand, and an MPhil in public administration from the University of Bergen, Norway. He earned his bachelor's and master's degrees from the University of Dhaka, Bangladesh. His research interests are human rights, healthcare, mental health, gender and sexuality, and social work issues.

Jacek Kolodziej completed a PhD at Massey University, Auckland, Aotearoa New Zealand, on the lived experiences of pre-exposure prophylaxis use in Aotearoa New Zealand. He holds a master's degree in psychology. His research interests revolve around HIV prevention and sexual health along with critical analysis of the cultural contexts and the epistemological underpinnings of accumulation of knowledge of human sexuality.

Kan Diana Kwok 郭勤 is Associate Professor in the Department of Special Education and Counselling, The Education University of Hong Kong. Diana was a social work educator with The Chinese University of Hong Kong and a social worker and mental health counsellor at schools and mental health services. Her current research interests include sexual and transgender prejudice, experiences of LGBTQIA+ youth, and school sexuality education. Her publications appear in the *Journal of Social Work Education, Children and Youth Services Review*, the *International Journal of Environmental Research and*

Public Health, *Qualitative Social Work*, *Sex Education*, the *International Review of Psychiatry* and the *Journal of LGBT Youth*, among others.

Barry Man Wai Lee 李文偉 is a guest lecturer in the Department of Special Education and Counselling at The Education University of Hong Kong. His primary areas of interest encompass masculinities, sexual health, sexual minorities and sexuality. Prior to joining academia, Lee was a senior social worker at the Hong Kong AIDS Foundation for over 14 years, working with people living with HIV/AIDS. Since 2014, Lee has also been a board member for Grey and Pride, a charitable organisation for older LGBTQ in Hong Kong, advocating and promoting social inclusion for the older LGBTQ community.

Tetyana Semigina is Professor at the Academy of Labour, Social Relations and Tourism, Ukraine, and a member of the National Qualification Agency. She has extensive experience working for various international projects. In 2011–16, Tetyana was a board member for the International Association of Schools of Social Work, serving as secretary. She has authored more than 400 publications on social work, social and health policy, and HIV/AIDS issues.

Michael Stevens has a Masters in Sociology and has been a freelance writer and commentator on the Aotearoa New Zealand Takatāpui/Rainbow communities for over 20 years. He has been living with HIV since 1988. He currently lives in Auckland with his fiancé and their greyhound, and works as a diversity and inclusion consultant.

Jacqui Stevenson is an HIV, sexual and reproductive health and rights and gender researcher and advocate with interest in feminist, participatory and creative research. Her PhD research at the University of Greenwich, UK, explored the experiences of older women living with HIV in London. She works internationally and nationally as a freelance consultant in research, training and advocacy promoting gender equality in the HIV response, and has served as a trustee of the Sophia Forum and STOPAIDS.

Yulia Stopolyanska is a physician and holds a Masters in Public Health Management from the School of Public Health, National University of Kyiv-Mohyla Academy, Ukraine. She has experience leading international projects to deliver quality care for viral hepatitis C and HIV/AIDS linked to accomplishing the UNAIDS 90-90-90 HIV and hepatitis C virus elimination targets. Additionally, she has comprehensive experience as a medical advisor in the pharmaceutical industry in Ukraine and abroad.

Tetiana Yurochko is Head of the School of Public Health, National University of Kyiv-Mohyla Academy, Ukraine. She has experience of working in international projects in the field of HIV/AIDS. In 2010–16, Tetiana worked at the National Institute for Strategic Studies of Ukraine and participated in the development of health policies in Ukraine.

Series editors' introduction

Paul Reynolds, Paul Simpson and Trish Hafford-Letchfield

This *Sex and Intimacy in Later Life* book series will explore, interrogate and enlighten upon the sensual, sexual and intimate lives of older people. The motivation for launching this series was a concern with the relative lack of attention in public, professional and academic/intellectual spheres to sex and intimacy in later life (indicatively, Hafford-Letchfield, 2008; Simpson et al, 2018a, 2018b). The series is intended to contribute to and enrich the development of the field of studies in the intersections of age, sex, sexuality and intimacy as a critical and important area of scholarship. It is only beginning to be recognised as an important social, cultural and political issue within and beyond the 'Western' academy, from which it has emerged. Its earliest contributions, of which this volume are a part, are motivated by a desire to recognise and reject the pathologies and prejudices that have infused this intersection – what Simpson has termed 'ageist erotophobia' (Simpson et al, 2018b, p 1479) – and fuels the failure to acknowledge older people as sexual agents. This is both an intellectual and a political agenda, to question and evaluate the impact of real rather than assumed losses of cognitive, physical, social and sexual capacity, and to recuperate older people as sexual agents from dismissal, ridicule and trivialisation.

If the latter half of the twentieth century was characterised by challenges to the pathologies of social identities – particularly gender, ethnicity and race, disability, sexuality – and struggles for recognition, rights and liberties, more intersectional struggles and recognitions characterise the twenty-first century (on intersectionality, see indicatively Hancock, 2016; Hill Collins and Bilge, 2016). Significant among these has been the re- evaluation of what it is to age and to be an older agent in contemporary societies. Older people have historically experienced both veneration and respect and neglect and pathology, largely based on differing cultural stereotypes of the value of age (Ylanne, 2012). The most common characterisation is that older people are not sexual, past being sexual or represent a problematic sexuality – or their sexuality is a superficial concern and secondary to concerns of health, care, life course and support by public services and engagement and pensions/ resources. Such concerns are those mainly of 'Western' cultures and reflected in the western influence across the globe in respect of state intervention and provision, but elsewhere they have been subsumed and often rendered invisible into family and kinship structures.

Older people's intimate and sexual lives and experiences have transformed in the last 40 years, as a consequence of a number of significant social changes: new technologies – digital, mechanical and pharmaceutical – and their interventions; the recognition of older people as exploitable markets for consumption; healthier lifestyles, changes and extensions to life course and life expectancy; the erosion of social and sexual pathologies around age and recognitions of different intersections and their importance (LGBTQI older people, older people of different ethnicities, older disabled/ neurodiverse and 'able- bodied/ minded' people; older men and women).[1] These transformations demonstrate evidence of increase in the sexual relations and intimacies of older people and their impacts, such as increased rates of STD transmission, or implications for healthy sex lives for older people in care institutions (indicatively, Drench and Losee, 1996; Lindau, 2007; Bodley-Tickell et al, 2008; Chao et al, 2011; Simpson, 2015; Age UK, 2019). The scholarship exploring these developments has only recently begun to catch up. A small but growing literature has focused on age and sexuality (represented in the sources authors draw from in this series), with a principal focus on the erosion of easy pathologies and stereotypes of older people's heteronormativity and heterosexuality. Particularly as the 'baby boomers' of the 1950s and 1960s move into old age, changed sexual attitudes, wants and needs require changed political, cultural and institutional responses. The older generation of baby boomers in the late 1940s and 1950s may have remembered Vera Lynn (an iconic British wartime singer singing patriotic songs during World War 2) and post- war society – retaining traditional stereotypes of older people. However, their horizons will have been formed and broadened more by influences from the 1960s' pop and rock culture (notably with such artists as the Beatles, Rolling Stones and Janis Joplin), women's and LGBT liberation struggles, the proliferation of accessible public representations of sex and the 'pornification' of society in the digital age.

Ageing and becoming 'older', intimacy, sexual identity, relations and practices, and sexual pleasure are all contested concepts and subject categories. They are understood as being constituted by different demarcations, distinctions and understandings arising from different intellectual disciplines, conceptual approaches, cultures, geographical credible to preclude critical and constructive debate on the meanings and demarcations of these intersections, it is necessary to draw some broad conceptual boundaries rather than hard- and- fast definitions. 'Ageing' and 'older' are broad categories that are attached to people considered in their 'third age' or 'later life' – in more

---

[1] One long, full version of what has been called the 'alphabet soup' of sexual identities is LGBTIQCAPGNGFNBA ('Lesbian', 'Gay', 'Bisexual', 'Transgender', 'Intersex', 'Questioning', 'Curious', 'Asexual', 'Pansexual', 'Gender Nonconforming', 'Gender-Fluid', 'Non-Binary' and 'Androgynous'). This list is extended in countries with cultural expressions of sexualities.

affluent countries/regions of the mainly Global North, the threshold is often seen as the age of 50+. This reflects common practice in the literatures of social gerontology, psychology and the sociology of ageing (see Zaninotto et al, 2009; Cronin and King, 2010; Stenner et al, 2011). It is after that, and into their sixth decade, that older people experience a process of de-eroticisation that could be called 'compulsory non- sexuality' (taking our cue from feminist theorist Adrienne Rich [1981], who articulated pressures on women's sexuality towards 'compulsory heterosexuality').

Ageing and being older can be understood mainly in two ways. First, the terms describe ageing as a chronological and physiological process involving key changes, which become particularly marked (and can be stigmatised) in the later stages of the life course. This raises questions around the differential impact of life course experience and physiological change – which may include loss and/ or reduction of physical and mental capacities for some people at different stages in the life course. It is structured both by physiological change and by the (often imperceptible) internalisation and normalisation of orthodoxies describing ageing and being older in cultural and social discourse, and everyday practice and experience of how older people are perceived and how older people see themselves – often as lacking – and in relation to younger people (Foucault, 1977, 1978). Such is the means by which older people (as much as younger people or social and cultural institutions) both produce and accept the discursive limits to ageing. Second, ageing and being older could be described as an attribution constituted by ideology and discourse, structural- hierarchical and cultural- discursive influences and material contexts, such as the structure of organisations, public spaces, cultural representations and spaces of connection (for example, labour markets). Ageing is usefully regarded as a product of intersections between the symbolic/ discursive and structural/ material dimensions of existence. The attribution of a particular age – young, mature or older – is an ideological construct suffused by power relations and composed of cultural attributions, instantiated in material processes and practices. These structural factors impose all manner of constraints on older people's sexual agency (though these can be questioned, challenged and resisted). Put simply, age is a social, cultural and political construct and how older people are perceived and valued – whether prejudicially or with respect – is constituted in the wider character of social values and dominant discourses. While age is an experienced and embodied phenomenon, its meaning is socially, culturally and politically mediated.

'Sex' and 'sexuality' are often distinguished by the former being focused on practices and behaviour, and the latter being focused on identities, relations and orientations. The terms are nevertheless porous and intertwined (Weeks, 2010). Sexuality describes the processes of being sexual (or not) in the world and through self- recognition, expressing (or not) sexual choices and preferences and enjoying (or not) sexual pleasures. It involves the expression of emotions, desires, beliefs, self- presentation and how we relate to others. It most commonly relates to sexual identity – for example hetero, lesbian, gay, bisexual, queer, asexual (Rahman and Jackson, 2010). Sexuality is multidimensional, being co- constituted by the biological (for example bodily sensations interpreted as 'sexual'), the psychological (for example emotions and reasoning) and cultural and socio- economic influences such as dressing up and flirting and so on (Doll, 2012). It is often understood narrowly as genitocentric, itself tied to the heteronormative relationship between genital sex and reproduction. Yet it encapsulates a range of practices that bring sensual pleasure and fulfil wants and desires, such as the agglomeration of practices that are subsumed under the umbrella term BDSM (indicatively Weiss, 2011; Ortmann and Sprott, 2013). 'Intimacy' refers to involvement in close and interpersonal relations. It can be a feature of diverse relationships, from those that are sexual, or with strong close personal friendship bonds, or characterised by physical and emotional closeness, to those where a particular relation or facet of life is shared closely, such as close work relationships. It encompasses a spectrum of emotions, needs and activities ranging from feelings of caring, closeness and affection (that can go with long- term companionship) through to 'romance', where an individual 'idealizes' a person(s) (Ehrenreich et al, 1997). Intimacy is to a degree conceived in gendered terms: if men tend to defi ne it more in physical terms, women usually emphasise more its emotional content (O'Brien et al, 2012). It is often conceived as two people sharing intimacy rather than a larger number and is constituted subjectively as a value that is owned or shared with others, although equally it is sometimes seen as an arena that reinforces oppressive conventions of private– public divides and 'compulsory monogamy' (Bersani and Phillips, 2008; Heckert, 2010; Musial, 2013).

These three conceptualisations – age/ older, sex/ sexuality and intimacies – intersect in complex ways. For example, the prevailing recognise 'fuck buddies' or so- called casual relationships for mutual sexual gratification (though intimacy is sometimes used to describe a particular event without relationship – 'they were intimate' (Wentland and Reissing, 2014). Likewise, sex and age often enmesh in complex ways, though these linkages too often involve mutually reinforcing negative representations. Decline in sexual capacity – often reduced to coital/ genital function – is associated with ageing and later life as a standard correlation as opposed to a graduated contingency. Drawing in other intersections, the relationship between sexual capacity and potency is a significant feature of masculinity and therefore sexual capacity is considered more challenging for men, given fears of loss of status and greater reluctance than women to seek help concerning sexual and relationship problems (O'Brien et al, 2012). This reflects gendered assumptions that male sexuality is more active and women's more passive that is rooted in classical sexology (indicatively Davidson and Layder,

1994; Bland and Doan, 1998). Nevertheless, the sexuality of older women could be constrained by biological changes, understood through cultural pathology as decline and loss of attractiveness. As female sexuality tends to be more associated with youth-coded beauty, older women become excluded from the sexual imaginary (Doll, 2012). In addition, women face the moral constraints of being a good wife/ mother/ grandmother, where being non- sexual is seen as a virtue and not a deficiency, whereby older women face moral censure for transgressing an approved ageing femininity when not acting their age (Lai and Hynie, 2011). As such the narrative of decline is perpetuated. Since the 1970s, however, women now over 50 will have encountered the countervailing influences of feminism and challenge such culturally constituted assumptions (Bassnett, 2012; Westwood, 2016).

Even where the idea of older sexual agents meets with approval because of its contribution to well- being and self- esteem, their sexuality has been subject to a medicalised, book- keeping approach that disregards emotions and pleasures and focuses on who is still 'doing it' (Gott, 2004), in the context of declining physical capacity for genitocentric penetrative sex (see Trudel, Turgeon and Piché, 2000, as an example). However, more encouragingly, we perceive the beginnings of challenge to these negative discourses in European, Australian and US contexts and writing, which attempt to recuperate older people, including the oldest citizens (commonly care home residents) and across the spectrum of genders and sexualities, as legitimate sexual/ intimate citizens (see Gott, 2004; Hafford-Letchfield, 2008; Bauer et al, 2012; Doll, 2012; Simpson et al, 2016, 2017; Villar et al, 2014). The purpose of elaborating these brief examples is to underline that a focus on sex and intimacy in later life involves the recognition of intersections both within and beyond the conceptual constituents of the series focus. Lives are not lived in sexual, intimate or aged based singularities, but in complex differentiated yet overlapping and intertwined experiences with myriad intersections, such as class, race/ethnicity, gender, disability, embodiment and affect (Simpson, 2015).

It is this rich patina of experience and knowledge creation that this series seeks to elucidate, working outward from a critical focus on the core concerns of sex/sexuality, intimacy and ageing, and providing the space for innovative and high- quality scholarship that can inform institutions, policy, professional practice, current and future research and older people experiencing this focus as lived experience and not simply subject of inquiry. The vision behind the series is that it will:

- put the sex back in sexuality (and into ageing). This arises from the observation that while sexuality studies has progressed considerably over the last 40 years (Fischer and Seidman, 2016), its development as an intellectual field of enquiry has to some extent dampened the subversive character of a focus on the 'messy physicality' of sexual pleasure. Put simply, there is lots of scholarship about sexuality, but less focus on the pleasures of sex. There is an aspiration that this series might be one avenue by which that can in a small way be corrected. Putting the 'sex' back into 'sexuality' is part of an agenda to recuperate older people to continue to be recognised as sexual citizens (or more specifically to have the choice to be sexual agents or not). As such, this series can support the vanguard of an intellectual project that will establish sex in later life as a serious yet neglected political issue and thus stimulate and advance debate. If what is at stake in understanding current experience is the impediments and constraints to choice and pleasure, embodied sensual practice and agency must constitute part of the site of scholarship;

- promote and offer an avenue for critically engaged work on the subject matter, whether it is empirical and theoretical- philosophical, from across the social sciences, humanities and cultural studies, incorporating scientific and aesthetic insights. An essential part of the project is that assumptions, claims and received knowledge about sex and intimacy in later life are always questioned, challenged and subject to critical review. This is the means by which both extant knowledge is tested, refined and strengthened or rejected, and new knowledge is produced. A critical frame also offers the opportunity to move beyond traditional academic frames – insofar as a book series allows – in presenting new ideas, evidence and conjectures;
- emphasise the value of multidisciplinary and interdisciplinary approaches to sex and intimacy in late life. Though the series is open to critical research studies from specific disciplinary positions, such as sociology, psychology or gerontology, it recognises the value of multi- disciplinary studies that draw on more than one discipline or field, and interdisciplinary studies that cut across and suture together different disciplines, perspectives and approaches in understanding the complexity of older people and their sexual and intimate lives. This extends to recognising the value of the interweaving of science, aesthetic and critical approaches across paradigm and disciplinary boundaries;
- recognise the value of different approaches that foreground the experiential and/ or empirical and/ or theoretical landscapes of sex and intimacy in later life, whether they form layered responses to a question or are presented as discrete levels of analysis;
- have an international focus, recognising global differences, inequalities; there is value in both the specificity and depth afforded regional, national and locally based studies but there should be acknowledgement of supranational, international and global contexts to phenomena, trends and developments and political, cultural and social responses. It should be acknowledged that the emergent knowledge on sex, intimacy and later life has been generated mostly within academies of the Global North, but it does not follow that this necessarily implies progress in comparison to

other parts of the globe. It also recognises that there are inherent difficulties of resourcing and organisational and common conceptualisation in the development of international projects with a global reach, and these difficulties are unevenly distributed across the globe. In some parts of the globe researching this focus is not simply difficult but inherently risky to those who might be researched or researched with through intolerance, hostility and lack of recognition. Genuine attempts at a global research agenda require properly distributed and balanced strategies for collaboration to meet relevant constraints and challenges. There should be both attention to the seeds of emergent scholarship in the Global South, and sensitivity to the tendency of western scholarship to reflect a bias towards a 'colonial' approach to knowledge production. Notwithstanding the tendency for scholarship to focus on the Global North and particularly North America, Europe and Australasia, the series seeks – in a small way– to promote international understandings. This is achieved through the conviction that cross- cultural and spatial perspectives, drawing from insight and evidence across the globe, can contribute to better understandings of experience and avenues for research, policy and practice and reflection;

- allow for language, labels and categories that emerge from partial geographical and cultural contexts in the development of scholarship to be questioned, adapted, resisted and brought into relief with alternatives and oppositions in how age, sex, sexuality and intimacy are conceived;
- recognise and explore the constraints on and complications involved in expression of sexual/ intimate citizenship as an older person and across a spectrum of sexual and gender identities, interrogating and challenging stereotypes of older people as prudish or sex- negative and post- sexual. Equally, the series seeks to explore, examine and advocate sex- positive approaches to sex and intimacy in later life that can help empower, enable and support older people's sexual and intimate relations;
- be accessible to readers in order to inform public understanding, academic study, intellectual debate, professional practice and policy development. This is an ambitious agenda to set for any enterprise, and the series hopes only to make modest contributions to it. Nevertheless, the series has been born of a conviction that unless this sort of agenda is adopted, the experience everyone shares of growing old will always be unnecessarily impoverishing and incapacitating. At the core of this series, and what it should exemplify, is the flourishing that arises from older sexual agents making choices, giving and enjoying pleasure and recognising options and experiences that are open to them as they age.

The Series Editors
October 2021

References

Age UK (2019) 'As STIs in older people continue to rise, Age UK calls to end the stigma about sex and intimacy in later life' [online], Available from: https://www.ageuk.org.uk/latest-press/articles/2019/october/as-stis-in-older-people-continue-to-rise-age-uk-calls-to-end-the-stigma-about-sex-and-intimacy-in-later-life/

Arber, S. and Ginn, J. (1995) '"Only connect": gender relations and ageing', in S. Arber and J. Ginn (eds) *Connecting Gender and Ageing*, Buckingham: Open University Press, pp 1–14.

Bassnett, S. (2012) *Feminist Experiences: The Women's Movement in Four Cultures*, London: Routledge.

Bauer, M., Fetherstonhaugh, D., Tarzia, L., Nay, R., Wellman, D. and Beattie, E. (2012) '"I always look under the bed for a man". Needs and barriers to the expression of sexuality in residential aged care: the views of residents with and without dementia', *Psychology and Sexuality*, 4(3): 296–309.

Bersani, L. and Phillips, A. (2008) *Intimacies*, Chicago, IL: Chicago University Press.

Bland, L. and Doan, L. (1998) *Sexology in Culture: Labelling Bodies and Desires*, Cambridge: Polity Press.

Bodley-Tickell, A.T., Olowokure, B.., Bhaduri, S., White, D.J., Ward, D., Ross, J.D.C., Smith, G., Duggal, H.V., and Gould, P. (2008) 'Trends in sexually transmitted infections (other than HIV) in older people: analysis of data from an enhanced surveillance system', *Sexually Transmitted Infections*, 84(4): 312–17.

Chao, J.-K., Lin, Y.-C., Ma, M.-C., Lai, C.-J., Ku, Y.-C., Kuo, W.-H. and Chao, I.-C. (2011) 'Relationship among sexual desire, sexual satisfaction and quality of life in middle-aged and older adults', *Journal of Sex and Marital Therapy*, 37(5): 386–403.

Cronin, A. and King, A. (2010) 'Power, inequality and identification: exploring diversity and intersectionality amongst older LGB adults', *Sociology*, 44(5): 876–92.

Davidson, J.O. and Layder, D. (1994) *Methods, Sex, Madness*, London: Routledge.

Doll, G.A. (2012) *Sexuality and Long-Term Care: Understanding and Supporting the Needs of Older Adults*, Baltimore, MD: Health Professions Press.

Drench, M.E. and Losee, R.H. (1996) 'Sexuality and the sexual capabilities of elderly people', *Rehabilitation Nursing*, 21(3): 118–23.

Ehrenfeld, M., Tabak, N., Bronner, G. and Bergman, R. (1997) 'Ethical dilemmas concerning the sexuality of elderly patients suffering from dementia', *International Journal of Nursing Practice*, 3(4): 255–9.

Fischer, N.L. and Seidman, S. (eds) (2016) *Introducing the New Sexuality Studies* (3rd edn), London: Routledge.

Foucault, M. (1977) *Discipline and Punish: The Birth of the Prison*, London: Penguin.

Foucault, M. (1978) *The History of Sexuality. Volume 1: An Introduction*, trans R. Hurley, Harmondsworth: Penguin.

Gott, M. (2004) *Sexuality, Sexual Health and Ageing*, London: McGraw-Hill Education.

Hafford-Letchfield, P. (2008) '"What's love got to do with it?" Developing supportive practices for the expression of sexuality, sexual identity and the intimacy needs of older people', *Journal of Care Services Management*, 2(4): 389–405.

Hancock, A.-M. (2016) *Intersectionality: An Intellectual History*, Oxford: Oxford University Press.

Heckert, J. (2010) 'Love without borders? Intimacy, identity and the state of compulsory monogamy', *The Anarchist Library* [online], Available from: https://theanarchistlibrary.org/library/jamie-heckert-love-with out-borders-intimacy-identity-and-the-state-of-compulsory-monogamy

Hill Collins, P. and Bilge, S. (2016) *Intersectionality*, Cambridge: Polity Press.

Lai, Y. and Hynie, M. (2011) 'A tale of two standards: an examination of young adults' endorsement of gendered and ageist sexual double standards', *Sex Roles*, 64(5–6): 360–71.

Lindau, S.T., Schumm, P., Laumann, E.O., Levinson, W., O'Muircheartaigh, C.A. and Waite, L.J. (2007) 'A study of sexuality and health among older adults in the United States', *New England Journal of Medicine*, 357(8): 762–74.

Musiał, M. (2013) 'Richard Sennett and Eva Illouz on the tyranny of intimacy: intimacy tyrannised and intimacy as a tyrant', *Lingua ac Communitas*, 23: 119–33.

O'Brien, K., Roe, B., Low, C., Deyn, L. and Rogers, S. (2012) 'An exploration of the perceived changes in intimacy of patients' relationships following head and neck cancer', *Journal of Clinical Nursing*, 21(17–18): 2499–508.

Ortmann, D. and Sprott, R. (2013) *Sexual Outsiders: Understanding BDSM Sexualities and Communities*, London: Rowman and Littlefield.

Rahman, M. and Jackson, S. (2010) *Gender and Sexuality: Sociological Approaches*, Cambridge: Polity Press.

Rich, A. (1981) *Compulsory Heterosexuality and Lesbian Experience*, London: Onlywomen Press.

Simpson, P. (2015) *Middle-Aged Gay Men, Ageing and Ageism: Over the Rainbow?* Basingstoke, UK: Palgrave Macmillan.

Simpson, P., Brown Wilson, C., Brown, L., Dickinson, T. and Horne, M. (2016) 'The challenges of and opportunities involved in researching intimacy and sexuality in care homes accommodating older people: a feasibility study', *Journal of Advanced Nursing*, 73(1): 127–37.

Simpson, P., Horne, M., Brown, L.J.E., Dickinson, T. and Torkington, K. (2017) 'Older care home residents, intimacy and sexuality', *Ageing and Society*, 37(2): 243–65.

Simpson, P., Almack, K. and Walthery, P. (2018a) '"We treat them all the same": the attitudes, knowledge and practices of staff concerning old/er lesbian, gay, bisexual and trans residents in care homes', *Ageing & Society*, 38(5): 869–99.

Simpson, P., Wilson, C.B., Brown, L.J., Dickinson, T. and Horne, M. (2018b) '"We've had our sex life way back": older care home residents, sexuality and intimacy', *Ageing & Society*, 38(7): 1478–501.

Stenner, P., McFarquhar, T. and Bowling, A. (2011) 'Older people and "active ageing": subjective aspects of ageing actively', *Journal of Health Psychology*, 16(3): 467–77.

Trudel, G., Turgeon, L. and Piché, L. (2000) 'Marital and sexual aspects of old age', *Sexual and Relationship Therapy*, 15(4): 381–406.

Villar, F., Celdrán, M., Fabà, J. and Serrat, R. (2014) 'Barriers to sexual expression in residential aged care facilities (RACFs): comparison of staff and residents' views', *Journal of Advanced Nursing*, 70(11): 2518–27.

Weeks, J. (2010) *Sexuality* (3rd edn), London: Routledge.

Weiss, M. (2011) *Techniques of Pleasure: BDSM and the Circuits of Sexuality*, Durham, NC: Duke University Press.

Wentland, J.J. and Reissing, E. (2014) 'Casual sexual relationships: identifying definitions for one-night stands, booty calls, fuck buddies and friends with benefits', *The Canadian Journal of Human Sexuality*, 23(3): 167–77.

Westwood, S. (2016) *Ageing, Gender and Sexuality: Equality in Later Life*, London: Routledge.

Ylanne, V. (ed) (2012) *Representing Aging: Images and Identities*, Houndmills, UK: Palgrave Macmillan.

Zaninotto, P., Falaschetti, E. and Sacker, A. (2009) 'Age trajectories of quality of life among older adults: results from the English Longitudinal Study of Ageing', *Quality of Life Research*, 18(10): 1301–9.

Foreword: Dare we hope for the erotic? HIV/AIDS, sexuality and ageing

OmiSoore H. Dryden

James R. Johnson Chair in Black Canadian Studies,
Faculty of Medicine
Interim Director, Black Studies in STEM Research Institute
Dalhousie University, Halifax, Nova Scotia

I engage in interdisciplinary scholarship and research that focuses on Black queer and trans people, significations of HIV/AIDS and restrictions on blood donations from Black diasporic communities in Canada. I am particularly interested in the social life of blood donation and how 'good' donors are imagined. Primarily I focus on how anti-Black homophobia/white supremacist heteropatriarchy undergirds much of how we understand a safe blood supply.

What has been revealed in this research is the ways in which sex phobia and the moralistic limits of sexual intimacy stand in for 'good' and 'effective' donor protocols. Blood, in this instance, becomes part of what Foucault (1990) identifies as the science of social control, where those deemed as high risk are positioned as not only a social dilemma but also a medical dilemma. There is also a collaboration between the medical (public health) community and the media to support the carrier/vector narrative of HIV and AIDS, with delimited purported 'high-risk' communities.

About four years ago, I was in a researcher meeting with Canadian Blood Services, the blood operator in Canada. I was the only Black researcher attending the meeting. A senior medical employee of Canadian Blood Services spoke about why asking behaviour-focused questions was inappropriate, stating that asking a 72-year-old grandmother the last time she had anal intercourse was beyond the pale. This white employee literally placed her hand to her throat, as if clutching pearls, to convey the seemingly impossibility of such a practice. I hold this moment alongside two others that speak reflexively about ageing and sex.

The first is a moment in Yvonne Welbon's (1999) biographical documentary, *Living with Pride: Ruth C. Ellis @100*, which recounts the life story of Ms Ruth Ellis as she celebrates her 100th birthday. Ruth Ellis was known at the time of her death as the oldest living Black lesbian. The film travels through various poignant moments of her life, providing an example of what old age could look like for queer and trans people. We see her attending dances, going camping, taking self-defence courses, visiting with friends and participating in political activism. It begs the questions: Will we be doing the same at her age? Will we be as active? The moment I want to highlight here – one of the numerous special moments of the film – is when Ruth is asked about the last time she had sex. Her answer: 95! Both the question and the answer represent the erotic, which Audre Lorde (2000) describes as 'a measure between the beginnings of our sense of self and the chaos of our strongest feelings. It is an internal sense of satisfaction to which, once we have experienced it, we know we can aspire' (p 54).

The second moment occurred in June 2016 when I had the great opportunity to speak with a group of Black lesbian, gay, bisexual and queer folks to explore the Black queer spaces created for community in the 1970s and 1980s in Toronto, Canada. Part of that conversation included reminiscences about HIV/AIDS, sex, sexual intimacies, death and loss. The moment that is relevant here is when Junior Harrison spoke about the moment he learned he was HIV-positive and how this diagnosis galvanised him into political action. Decades later, he continued to feel the loss of all who died. He stated in our interview at the time:

> It's true, we talk about it all the time. My brothers. … There's a group, the AIDS generation, who would have been in their forties to fifties today, but they are gone. So when I go out, those few times I do, into Black gay spaces, I'm with men in their twenties and thirties, but not their forties or fifties. (Junior Harrison, interviewee quoted in Dryden, 2018, p 72)

It may seem inappropriate to speak about sexual intimacy and death simultaneously; however, these are the very moments to consider these interconnected intimacies. In our later discussions regarding the deployment of 'slut shaming', we reflected on how our sexualities and sexual practices – including BDSM (bondage, discipline, sadism and masochism), polyamory, non-monogamy, sex parties, bathhouses, dungeons – are policed. Exploring our full erotic pleasure – before HIV/AIDS, at the height of the pandemic and after – brings disapproval.

This type of stigma has resulted in a cataloguing of us into acceptable and unacceptable sexual groupings. Sexually based stigma results in homophobia and transphobic discrimination that facilitates increased health disparities and poorer health outcomes. Stigma and discrimination reflect the many ways that sexuality is regulated and under increased surveillance, thus animated within health settings. Forced (hyper)invisibility causes harm by undermining our health and well-being. We call it 'stigma', but it is the impact of racism, homophobia, transphobia, cisgenderism and misogyny. These types of respectability politics, which are used to frame the correct way to exist in normative and restrictive societies, ultimately serve to further the harm we experience in our lives.

HIV/AIDS has had a global impact in our communities. International and nationally funded HIV programmes have structured sexuality within biopolitical public health regulations. Sexual exceptionalism and homonormativity work to occlude the very inequalities in our various locations that exacerbate stigma and thus place us at greater risk for transmission and introduce greater struggle for health management. HIV/AIDS is understood as an epidemic on multiple simultaneous levels: it is an epidemic of a transmissible lethal disease as well as an epidemic of meanings or significations (Treichler, 1999). The signification of HIV/AIDS involves the stickiness of the systems of homophobia, racism and unknown blood-borne disease; and this stickiness is defined by Ahmed (2004) as 'a form of relationality' (p 91).

Effectively addressing and confronting stigma and health disparities requires a commitment to intersectionality in both method and modes of thought. Intersectionality, in this discourse, identifies the relationships between health stigma and systems of oppression, including how structures of stereotyping essentialise HIV, sexuality and sexual intimacies. Stereotyping animates the normative divides between what is deemed acceptable and unacceptable. There is a fixity to this practice of stereotyping that ostracises what doesn't belong, or that which unbelongs.

As one ages, it is assumed that our desire abates and our sexual intimacy is no longer required. Yet, to believe this is to truncate the fullness of our stories. Queer and trans people living as older people is more than just a possibility for many with HIV/AIDS, and it is important and necessary that we explore the nuances of the assemblages of our erotic selves.

What does it mean to both imagine growing older with HIV/AIDS and continue to engage in sexual intimacy? *HIV, Sex, and Sexuality in Later Life* brings these moments together, highlighting various experiences from across the globe. It re-narrates the ways in which we animate our lives, thus bringing us a bit closer to the full exploration of the (our) erotic.

The contributors in this book examine and use empirical research, autoethnography and personal stories to document and explore our diverse, complicated and incoherent lives. They provide insight into how to manage being positioned as unruly, uncivil and outside of the norm. They demonstrate the richness of possibility available to us in disrupting normative structures of health, wellness, sexuality, intimacy and ageing. The concept of health must take into account physical, psychological and social well-being.

The links between sexuality and power inform not only how we understand our own sexual lives, but also how we operate within the significations of HIV/AIDS. In this collection, the authors demonstrate that by refusing the silencing of our desires and by speaking them aloud (at least to ourselves), perhaps we are able to bring our sexual intimacies into our futures as we age. In this way, we are able to disrupt the continuing social stigmas of HIV/ AIDS and homophobia/transphobia, and their attendant harms. As Patricia Hill Collins (2004) states:

> Sexual contact constitutes one main source of HIV infection. Because sexual intimacy reflects an individual's relationship with his or her own body as well as how others see and value that body, individual sex acts are highly politicised. The danger posed by HIV/AIDS forces individual men and women to weigh the nature of each sexual contact, as well as all interpersonal relationships in which sexual expression might take physical form. (p 289)

As queer and trans people and people of colour, we are often blamed for our own problems. Black people, queer and trans communities and communities of colour are blamed, and perceived as being immorally sexually promiscuous and thus responsible for bringing disease and death, not to 'their' communities but to the 'general public'.

As argued in the afterword of this book, the gaze needs to shift from marginalised communities towards the systems that perpetuate harmful stigma and continuing marginalisation. Sexually transmitted blood-borne infections are a reality, occurring throughout society. What facilitates poorer outcomes and death are the ways in which sexually transmitted and blood-borne infections are framed as a moral failing, a lack of virtue, something to be ashamed about. This prevents us from seeking treatment and support, fearing that we will be judged and made to feel responsible for the transmission of disease. By shifting the gaze to systems of marginalisation, barriers to care are reduced and supports for greater quality of life are increased.

Overall, these chapters capture what it means to speak about our gender and sexuality, our HIV status and sexual pleasure. Our sexualities continue to generate controversy in relation to how we age, as we still grapple with the belief that sex is only for reproduction and any other sexual practice is immoral. And this is especially visited on post-menopausal persons who continue to engage in sexual activities that bring and centre pleasure. Our collective histories of gender and sexuality become occluded through puritanical indoctrination, imperial advertising and neoliberal logics of respectability.

What we learn in this collection are the ways in which stigma, respectability politics and significations of HIV/AIDS continue to steal from the fullness of our lives. But we also learn about how people are embracing the erotic, in its fullest sense, in their lives. We are ageing. And for some this is an unexpected and pleasant surprise – something we didn't think would or could happen. And by ageing, we are now living lives we didn't dare imagine and/or hope for.

References

Ahmed, S. (2004) *The Cultural Politics of Emotion*, Edinburgh: Edinburgh University Press.

Dryden, O. (2018) 'Má-ka Juk Yuh: a genealogy of Black queer liveability in Toronto', in J. Haritaworm, G. Moussa and S.M. Ware with R. Rodríguez (eds) *Queering Urban Justice: Queer of Colour Formations in Toronto*, Toronto: University of Toronto Press, pp 62–83.

Foucault, M. (1990) *The History of Sexuality. Volume 1: An Introduction*, trans R. Hurley, New York: Vintage Books.

Hill Collins, P. (2004) *Black Sexual Politics: African Americans, Gender, and the New Racism*, New York: Routledge.

Lorde, A. (2000) *Uses of the Erotic: The Erotic as Power*, Tucson, AZ.: Kore Press.

Treichler, P.A. (1999) *How to Have Theory in an Epidemic: Cultural Chronicles of AIDS*, Durham, NC: Duke University Press.

Welbon, Y. (dir) (1999) *Living with Pride: Ruth Ellis @ 100* [film], Chicago, Our Film Works.

Introduction

*Mark Henrickson, Casey Charles, Shiv Ganesh, Sulaimon Giwa,
Kan Diana Kwok and Tetyana Semigina*

This book would have been unimaginable 35 years ago.

And yet, here we are. That, perhaps, is the central, unifying theme to this volume: all kinds of people living with HIV are alive, growing older and seeking to live all of their lives, including their sexual selves.

The world has been distracted by a different pandemic over the last few years, and certainly the readily transmissible COVID-19 has presented a major threat to the world and the global health infrastructure. But COVID-19 is far more promiscuous than HIV/AIDS about people it infects, which means stigma against people living with the coronavirus has been very limited, and protests have been more against government regulation and interventions than people with the coronavirus. The global health community, while arguably not in a timely enough way, moved with remarkable speed for such bureaucratic organisations. With a few notable exceptions, government responses to COVID-19 have been unprecedentedly rapid and robust. These responses have been far different from government responses to AIDS in the earliest days, when AIDS was called 'GRID' (1982, Gay-Related Immune Deficiency) in the United States, and from the refusal for years of some governments to acknowledge HIV in their countries (Boone and Batsell, 2001; Chigwedere et al, 2008; King, 2021). UNAIDS (2021) estimates that nearly 38 million people were living with HIV in 2020; since the start of the epidemic in the late 1970s, 79.3 million have been infected with HIV and 36.3 million have died from AIDS-related illnesses. Most of those infected and affected by HIV were in already-stigmatised communities: people in poor countries, poor people in wealthy countries, people of colour, men who have sex with men, injection drug users and combinations of all of these. The intersecting diseases of virus, stigma, fear, racism and discrimination greatly impeded the development of care for people living with HIV. It is notable that, because of the tremendous research foundation laid in the search for HIV treatments and vaccines, vaccines for COVID-19 were produced with unprecedented speed (Zuckerman and McKay, 2020).

The editors and contributors to this book have decades of experience of living with HIV or working with people living with HIV. The idea of writing about the lives of older people living with HIV for much or most of their lives would have been unthinkable in the earliest years of the epidemic. At the height of the epidemic, many of us woke each morning dreading the news the day would bring of yet more deaths, or wondering what new hell the virus (or its treatments) would enact on our bodies. Yet somehow we are all here. Research, new technologies and simple dogged refusal to die has meant that more and more people are living longer and longer lives with HIV, even in places where these technologies are scarce or difficult to access. It is not just that people are diagnosed with HIV at young ages and are living longer, of course; as people continue to be sexually active throughout their entire lives, some people are diagnosed with HIV in later life. The biosociality of HIV has changed. Yet prevention technologies – technologies which prevent transmission, prevent disease progression and prevent death – are insufficient to overcome fears of stigma and rejection, and they also bring new challenges with them.

It has long been acknowledged that there is no age limit on sexual responsiveness or the need for intimacy and that sexuality and intimacy contribute to the quality of life of older persons (Benbow and Beeston, 2012). Although intimacy and sexuality are an integral part of human identity (Elias and Ryan, 2011), ageist, erotophobic assumptions define older people as post-sexual and exclude them from what has been called 'sexual citizenship' (Simpson et al, 2017). Older adults who do not have intimate relationships are often lonely and socially isolated, and at risk for an array of well-being issues (Victor et al, 2009; Malcolm et al, 2019). We are beginning to understand how different generations, population cohorts and cultures have very different understandings and expectations of sexuality and sexual activity (Aggleton et al, 2012; Peluso et al, 2012). Older people today challenge so-called traditional notions of sexuality and the hegemony of penetrative sex; it is health status rather than age that impacts sexuality (Gewirtz-Meydan et al, 2019), yet few providers feel prepared to respond to older adult sexuality (Hughes and Wittmann, 2015). While sexual identity should be included in any comprehensive assessment of a client trying to access social services or of a patient (Hughes, 2003), few providers do so (Neville and Henrickson, 2006). As people live longer, support for older persons with their sexual lives by knowledgeable providers will become increasingly important (Træen et al, 2017).

This book is an edited anthology of all kinds of experiences of people living with HIV around the world. In style it is an eclectic collection of different sorts of writing – empirical research, personal reflection, poetry and mixtures of these – because there is no single kind of writing that can capture the multifarious, intersectional experiences of older people living with HIV. The editors of this volume have a variety of disciplinary backgrounds, mainly social work but also communications and literature. Contributors also come from a wide array of disciplinary backgrounds and personal experiences. They consider the experiences of Swiss women living in 'sexual retirement' (not always by choice), women in Ukraine, Black African migrant women in the United Kingdom, gay men in Aotearoa New Zealand, Italy and the United Kingdom rediscovering their sexual selves and intimate relationships as a result of medication technologies, Hong Kongese gay and bisexual men living with HIV, gender and sexually diverse South Asians and Black African women and men living with HIV in Kenya. The only things that all of these diverse peoples have in common is HIV, and their experiences of stigma, despair, determination and possibility that they have lived over the past several decades.

The present volume is the third in a planned series of five on sexuality in later life, and we hope that you will find other volumes in this series useful and engaging. One of the things we have recognised in preparing this book is that 'later life' is very much a relative term. It is relative not only for individuals, but also in the context of their cultures and societies. While in developed nations, later life may refer to being over the age of 50, in poorer nations with multiple health and social challenges, it may refer to being over 30. Since we have been deliberately very international in our approach, we have been very flexible in our understanding of later life. Poverty challenges our notions of the length, expectations and quality of life. What is normal in one national setting may be unimaginable in another. We invite the reader to approach this volume with an open mind as well as an open heart. In places where new HIV treatments, such as antiretroviral therapies and pre-exposure prophylaxis (PrEP), are readily available, these have transformed the physical and social experience of HIV and sexuality. It is these technologies that have made this book both possible and necessary.

Two groups affected by HIV – heterosexual women and gay men – have very different experiences of these technologies. Older heterosexual women appear reluctant to re-engage with sexuality even when their viral loads are suppressed to undetectable levels. Gay men, however, reclaim their sexuality with enthusiasm. In her study of the trajectories of 30 older women living with HIV in Switzerland, Vanessa Fargnoli reminds us that in the first instance sexuality related to 'older' people, with or without HIV, is considered taboo and is a topic of minimal interest. These research and practice blind spots exist because ageist stereotypes are embedded in contemporary gender and sexual norms. So-called traditional understandings of women's sexuality are focused on reproduction, which creates a kind of biological determinism; women who do not or cannot reproduce are not valued. HIV undermines values that are embedded in heteronormative discourses that construct women mostly as mothers, nurturers, wives, carers and also virtuous and romantic lovers. Participants in Fargnoli's study spoke about their common experiences of dangerous bodies – that is, bodies with HIV. Even though contemporary medical treatments that render viral loads undetectable (and therefore HIV non-transmissible) have changed this understanding of the dangerous body, these women still talked about sexual retirement.

It is the technologies themselves that shape the focus of Jacqui Stevenson's chapter on the biomedicalisation of health in people living with HIV. Biomedicalisation is defined as the extension of medical jurisdiction so that it is concerned with not merely with illness and disease but also health more broadly. Women who are long-term survivors of HIV struggle to plan for and negotiate an older age they never expected to reach, and recently diagnosed older women face challenges as they negotiate older age with an unexpected HIV diagnosis. The 18 women who took part in body mapping workshops as part of Stevenson's study, mostly (but not exclusively) Black African migrants to the United Kingdom, reported a multifaceted conception of stigma, both internalised and enacted externally, that intersected with other forms of discrimination, including sexism, ageism, racism, anti-migrant discrimination and anti-trans discrimination. The was no unitary or single experience of HIV and ageing among this group, but the experiences of living with HIV and ageing were intersectional. These women also described sex as something out of reach or no longer desired.

Tetyana Semigina, Tetiana Yurochko and Yulia Stopolyanska employed a structuralist perspective to understand the specifics of stigma experienced by nine older women living with HIV in pre-war Ukraine. They found that healthy ageing requires specific, tailored education for people as they age and that this education needs to be not only about HIV but also about the sexual lives of older persons. Older women, especially older women living with HIV, are invisibilised. Like their counterparts in other nations, older women in Ukraine reported difficulty re-engaging sexually after their diagnosis with HIV, even if they had undetectable viral loads. Some of these women deliberately restricted or avoided sexual intercourse because of their conscious fear of infecting a sexual partner. Others reported not feeling any sexual desire. A trusting relationship between women and their medical providers is essential, but these researchers found instead that these older women living with HIV were wary of discussing their sexual lives with their physicians.

In the United Kingdom and Italy, Cesare Di Feliciantonio interviewed 25 gay men living with HIV who participate in chemsex – that is, the use of drugs such as GHB, GHL, crystal methamphetamine and mephedrone to enhance and facilitate sex. He found that participants framed their engagement with chemsex as driven by the quest for sociality combined with a rediscovery of sexual pleasure and an improved sense of comfort with their bodies resulting from the emergence of the paradigm of undetectability. He also found ambivalences and tensions within participants' engagement with chemsex. In order to fully understand the relationship between chemsex and the life course for older gay men living with HIV, it is necessary to consider both intergenerationality and intersectionality.

PrEP also plays an important role in recovering the joy and intimacy of sexual encounters among those whose lives have been impacted by the generational experience of HIV. Jacek Kolodziej presents the case study of Allan, an older White gay man in Aotearoa New Zealand. Allan describes how the history of HIV maps onto the trajectory of his sexual life. PrEP underlined dramatic shifts in his HIV prevention practices. In allowing Allan to be sexually active with other gay men again, PrEP became an agent of transformation that replaced the difficult emotions of grief and loss associated with HIV with those of joy, pleasure and feelings of connectedness to other men. Allan uses the metaphor of peeling away the layers to describe this process of reconnection, which suggests that these layers are the residue of living with a fear of HIV that was distorting connections with other men and gay communities. It is medical prevention technologies which now allow Allan to re-engage enthusiastically with his sexuality and with the wider gay community.

In his autoethnography, writer Michael Stevens recounts the sexual experiences of his youth and describes feeling like his world had ended when he discovered his HIV diagnosis, sex being fraught and dangerous as he lived with HIV, and then rediscovering intimacy and physical connection in his relationship in later life. 'I have long believed the thing that really makes us gay' he writes, 'is our desire to fully love and be loved by the same sex, not just the sex acts themselves. Now that I have that love and intimacy in my life, sex has receded in importance.' For Stevens, intimacy has replaced sexual activity as a focus of later life. Treatments for HIV have restored choice to his sexuality: 'Now it is something again that is not what it was, something that still always carries a shadow, but can, if I wish it, return to something close to the freedom and ecstasy I so enjoyed in my youth.' 'Today it feels an incidental part of our relationship and who we are together.'

Barry Man Wai Lee reminds us that older Chinese gay and bisexual men in Hong Kong, like their heterosexual counterparts, are not an homogeneous group. Early life experiences of being socially outcast and criminalised, and male homosexuality being classified as a mental illness are part of their shared common histories. Four overarching themes emerged from their experiences of sexuality, HIV and ageing: being different (from the 'ideal' of heterosexuality); experiencing subtle and indirect harassment, or what we might call today microaggressions; trying to fulfil filial and social obligations of getting married to a women while secretly exploring same-sex desires; the double stigma of living with HIV and as gay/bisexual men in heterosexual marriages; and reaffirming their sexuality as they aged and reconstructed their self-identified sexualities. Here, medical technologies played only a small role in the ways these men lived their older lives.

In his part autoethnographic, part poetic and part empirical piece, writer Casey Charles struggles with the right to interview and to make meaning across cultural boundaries, and answers his own question: 'What right had I, [an HIV] positive writer landing in Nairobi in 2009, *not* to seek out the stories of others growing older with the pandemic?' He makes the salient point that age is a relative notion, noting that the life expectancy of a person living with HIV in sub-Sharan Africa is 54, and in some regions as low as 49. Here, later life begins much earlier than in developed nations. In this chapter we encounter the author's experiences of living with HIV and the stories of Kenyans he meets, in particular Jane E, a woman of around 40 who is living with HIV and who had become instrumental in her community by providing information and hope to other people living with HIV. Once again we encounter experiences of stigma and are reminded of important intersectional and intercultural experiences of a community of people living with HIV. In this chapter it is not the experiences of medical technologies or of sexuality that creates community, but HIV itself.

Kanamik Kani Khan focuses his attention on the story of Didi, a 60-something Muslim lesbian living in urban Bangladesh. She describes her struggles with depression associated with the social stigma of being different in a society that is highly heterosexualised and gender-conforming – at least to outward appearances. Didi's story stands in for the stories of gender and sexually marginalised people in Bangladesh and their experiences of relationships and access to healthcare. By exploring her difference, Didi discovered her resilience, and this helped her to become an advocate for gender and sexually diverse communities, even representing those communities alongside the government bodies that once oppressed her.

Casey Charles makes a reappearance in his chapter about Sanjeevani, a community organisation created to support gender and sexually diverse people in Mumbai. In the context of a society where access to HIV medications and the ability to adhere to medication regimens is extraordinarily challenging, we are once again reminded that later life is a very relative concept. These challenges come not only from poverty, although that is the backdrop on which these stories are lived, but from the social structures and expectations that are imposed and lived in India. HIV is only one of an array of health and social challenges experienced by the people Charles interviews. The question he raises for us here is what kind of life has emerged for long-term survivors of HIV who 'suffer from early-onset ageing – physically, socially even psychologically' – people who live with herpes, hepatitis, tuberculosis and other chronic conditions as well as loneliness, isolation and depression.

HIV has always been more than a medical diagnosis. It is a social diagnosis born of poverty, stigma, discrimination and multiple oppressions. It has brought out the best in all kinds of health and social research and practice, but also brings the worst aspects of societies and cultures into sharp focus. As we move into what we might think of as the third era of HIV, it is appropriate once again to consider how we think about HIV and people living with HIV, how we think about ageing and how we think about sex and intimacy. Certainly, there is no single 'right' way to think about any of these things, but there are ways that are hurtful, stigmatising and destructive. Responsible health and social care workers will want to learn how to care for older people living with HIV and to support them to live all of their lives in the fullest possible way. This means, once again, challenging our assumptions, particularly about ageing and sexuality, and renewing our commitment to advocate and work for more socially just and inclusive societies.

As proud as we are of our recruitment of international contributors and experiences in this volume, we acknowledge that there are notable gaps in this work. There are no contributions from Indigenous and Indigenous African authors, and there is a wide gap in the Latin American experiences. We attempted to recruit widely through our international networks. While writing in English may have presented a barrier to some contributors, the silence in these spaces may reflect silence around HIV, sexuality, and HIV and sexuality in some cultures and societies. We hope this volume will present both an opportunity and a challenge to researchers, writers and practitioners in these regions to begin to talk about the unspeakable, to break the stigma and silence that continues to surround HIV and sexuality in some places.

References

Aggleton, P., Boyce, P., Moore, H.L. and Parker, R. (eds) (2012) *Understanding Global Sexualities: New Frontiers*, New York: Routledge.

Benbow, S.M. and Beeston, D. (2012) 'Sexuality, aging and dementia', *International Psychogeriatrics*, 24(7): 1026–33.

Boone, C. and Batsell, J. (2001) 'Politics and AIDS in Africa: research agendas in political science and international relations', *Africa Today*, 48(2): 3–22.

Chigwedere, P., Seage, G.R., Gruskin, S., Lee, T.-H. and Essex, M. (2008) 'Estimating the lost benefits of antiretroviral drug use in South Africa', *Journal of Acquired Immune Deficiency Syndrome*, 49(4): 410–15.

Elias, J. and Ryan, A. (2011) 'A review and commentary on the factors that influence expressions of sexuality by older people in care homes', *Journal of Clinical Nursing*, 20(11–12): 1668–76.

Gewirtz-Meydan, A., Hafford-Letchfield, T., Ayalon, L., Benyamini, Y., Biermann, V., Coffey, A., Jackson, J., Phelan, A., Voß, P., Zeman, M.G. and Zeman, Z. (2019) 'How do older people discuss their own sexuality? A systematic review of qualitative research studies', *Culture, Health & Sexuality*, 21(3): 293–308.

Hughes, A.K. and Wittmann, D. (2015) 'Aging sexuality: knowledge and perceptions of preparation among U.S. primary care providers', *Journal of Sex & Marital Therapy*, 41(3): 304–13.

Hughes, M. (2003) 'Talking about sexual identity with older men', *Australian Social Work*, 56(3): 258–66.

King, N. (2021) '40 years later: the denialism that shaped the AIDS epidemic', *NPR* [online], 18 May, Available from: https://www.npr.org/2021/05/18/ 997783457/40-years-later-the-denialism-that-shaped-the-aids-epidemic

Malcolm, M., Frost, H. and Cowie, J. (2019) 'Loneliness and social isolation causal association with health-related lifestyle risk in older adults: a systematic review and meta-analysis protocol', *Systematic Reviews* [online], 8: 48. doi: 10.1186/s13643-019-0968-x

Neville, S. and Henrickson, M. (2006) 'Perceptions of lesbian, gay and bisexual people of primary healthcare services', *Journal of Advanced Nursing*, 55(4): 407–15.

Peluso, P.R., Watts, R.E. and Parsons, M. (eds) (2012) *Changing Aging, Changing Family Therapy*, New York: Routledge.

Simpson, P., Horne, M., Brown, L.J.E., Wilson, C.B., Dickinson, T. and Torkington, K. (2017) 'Old(er) care home residents and sexual/intimate citizenship', *Ageing & Society*, 37(2): 243–65.

Træen, B., Hald, G., Graham, C., Enzlin, P., Janssen, E., Kvalem, I., Carvalheira, A. and Štulhofer, A. (2017) 'Sexuality in older adults (65+)— an overview of the literature, part 1: sexual function and its difficulties', *International Journal of Sexual Health*, 29(1): 1–10.

UNAIDS (2021) 'Global HIV & AIDS statistics—fact sheet' [online], Available from: https://www.unaids.org/en/resources/fact-sheet

Victor, C., Scambler, S. and Bond, J. (2009) *The Social World of Older People: Understanding Loneliness and Isolation in Later Life*, Maidenhead, UK: Open University Press.

Zuckerman, G. and McKay, B. (2020) 'How HIV research laid the foundation for Covid vaccines', *The Wall Street Journal* [online], 24 December, Available from: https://www.wsj.com/articles/how-hiv-research-laid-the-foundat ion-for-covid-vaccines-11608821508

PART I

Women

1

The 'disease of love': trajectories of women ageing with HIV in Switzerland

Vanessa Fargnoli

Introduction

More than 40 years have passed since the first cases of AIDS were reported in 1981. The apocalyptic scenario of the 1980s was replaced by an optimistic medical discourse following the advent of antiretroviral therapy (ART). ART transformed HIV into a manageable public health issue (Rosenbrock et al, 2000; World Health Organization, 2016) and increased the life expectancy of people living with HIV in high-income countries (Hasse et al, 2011). The ageing of people living with HIV, referred to as the ' "graying" of the epidemic' (Blanco et al, 2010, p 218), is gaining recognition (High et al, 2012; Banens et al, 2015). It raises several questions among HIV/AIDS experts and people living with HIV, especially as regards medical issues such as comorbidities and care services dependency (Kearney et al, 2010; Levett et al, 2014). While the life expectancy of people living with HIV is increasing, new HIV-positive diagnoses among people aged 50 and over are also rising (Banens et al, 2015; Bernard et al, 2018). Beyond medical and health-related concerns, few studies report on the social experiences of ageing with HIV in high-income countries. In the rare cases that do, women are under-represented or continue to be classified as 'others' (Mensah, 2003; Banens et al, 2015). In effect, in the official history of the AIDS epidemic, women living with HIV have been forgotten in clinical, epidemiological and social science research (Corea, 1993; Wilton, 1997; Mensah, 2003; Webel et al, 2013), except for women considered at risk of transmitting the virus, such as sex workers (Treichler, 1987), migrants (Poglia Mileti et al, 2014), mothers (Latham et al, 2001) and caregivers (McIntosh and Rosselli, 2012). However, not all women living with HIV fit into these categories.

In Switzerland, which is characterised by a liberal model of public health, approximately 20,000 people are living with HIV. Women make up a quarter of this population. While men are mainly infected through sexual relations with other men, women are mostly (70 per cent) infected through heterosexual intercourse (FOPH, 2018b). The key HIV populations defined by the Federal Office of Public Health (FOPH) are: homosexual men and men having sex with men, drug users, sex workers and people from countries with a high HIV prevalence (FOPH, 2018a).[1] Women who do not belong to these target groups have historically been ignored and are absent from medical and public debates about HIV/AIDS (Fargnoli, 2021).

To fill this double gap —women living with HIV and the sexuality of 'older' women – I use this chapter to discuss how ageing with HIV can affect women's sexuality and love lives. In the first section, I introduce two frames of reference: 'older' women's sexuality, and gender and sexual norms. These frames shape social, gender and sexual representations that affect women's lives. In the second section, I present experiences of women ageing with HIV in the French-speaking part of Switzerland.

Sex has an age and a gender

Gender and sexual orientations have profoundly shaped the medical and social representations of the AIDS epidemic. Sexuality related to 'older' people, with or without HIV, is considered 'taboo' (Lusti-Narasimhan and Beard, 2013, p 707), a 'topic of minimal interest' or a 'blind spot' (Saka et al, 2019, and Aboderin, 2014, cited in Banke-Thomas et al, 2020). Ageist stereotypes are also embedded in gender and sexual norms.

'Older' women's sexual frame

In Western countries, women's sexualities have been medically and socially constructed according to their 'biological clock' (Shorter, 1984; Ruault, 2015). Due to biomedical norms (obstetrics and gynaecology, and biotechnologies), the sexual lives of women are 'utero–centred' and 'programmed' according to a gendered temporal model following sequences related to procreation and female heterosexuality. They are expected to undergo successive sexual stages from 'voluntary infertility followed by a time dedicated to procreation, itself interrupted by infertile phases, then a new time of infertility that is socially obligatory, which precedes biological infertility (menopause)' (Ruault, 2015, p 44). According to Ruault (2015), discrimination related to age is rooted in obstetrics and gynaecology practices that define sexual identities and sexual boundaries according to stages of life that are both biologically and socially defined. Women's sexualities are trapped in a 'biological determinism', rooted in the medical and gynaecological cultures where motherhood is the core model of the female life and menopause as the cessation of all sexual activities. In contrast, a

---

[1] Quotes from French-language sources have been translated into English by the author.

biological clock is not imposed on men's sexualities, since medicine does not intervene on them. As Ruault (2015) argues further, 'they are told that they are not as old, that they retain (for longer) an insensitivity to old age' (p 48).

'Older' women are sexually and socially represented as asexual, without sexual desires and needs (Lusti-Narasimhan and Beard, 2013), and their aged bodies are presented as dysfunctional or undesirable (Lagrave, 2011; Ruault, 2015). Indeed, the ageing body means also a body more prone to diseases rooted in the biomedical construction of women's bodies as vulnerable, fragile or pathological (Shorter, 1984; Wilton, 1997; Ruault, 2015). As highlighted by Lagrave (2011), some argue that the renunciation of sexuality develops in parallel with ageing; they see 'a sort of equation between the ageing of the body and the decline of desire and sexual impulses. Sexuality would desert bodies that are undesirable because they are old' (p 2).

Therefore, as women age, sexual issues are addressed mainly from a clinical perspective. Menopause is perceived as requiring medical interventions (Banke-Thomas et al, 2020) and as putting an end to women's sexual lives (Lusti-Narasimhan and Beard, 2013; Ruault, 2015). This sexual frame for 'older' women is also rooted in gender and sexual norms.

Gender and sexual norms

Gender norms construct women in social roles as mothers, wives, carers and nurturers (Héritier, 2013), mainly in caring roles (Kergoat, 2005). These traditional representations establish a normative framework producing gender role assignments: women are expected to perform their priority roles as wives and mothers. If they fail to do so, they are criticised (Kergoat, 2005).

As with gender roles, men's and women's sexual roles have been socially constructed in different ways. For women, 'normal' expectations in relation to sexuality are heterosexual, passive, romantic, sentimental, monogamous, modest, serious, moral, faithful and non-adventurous (Dorlin, 2005; Mottier, 2008). On the other hand, men's sexuality is constructed as risky, active, powerful, adventurous, impulsive and involving multiple partners (Bajos and Bozon, 2008; Brenot and Wunsch, 2016). In addition, sexual health messages are mainly targeted at heterosexual women, who are assigned responsibility within couples for protecting sexual health and using contraception (Campbell, 1995; Mottier, 2008). This gender division – 'affective sexuality' for women and 'impulsive sexuality' for men – constructs male sexuality as being more important, with men having needs that must be satisfied.

However, HIV infection challenges these patterns and perceptions. Among men, HIV infection leads to the suspicion of homosexuality, a transgression of the heterosexual norm. For women, HIV undermines traditional family values embedded in heteronormative norms considering women mostly as mothers, nurturers, wives, carers and virtuous and romantic lovers (Théry, 1999; Héritier, 2013). As highlighted by Mensah (2003): 'What distinguishes the situation of women [with HIV] from that of gay men relates to the socially imposed roles of women, such as sexual availability to their partners, responsibility for protection in sexual relationships, the non-transmission of the virus to newborns, and care of children and relatives' (p 34). Indeed, many authors argue that HIV affects women's gender and sexual roles (Théry, 1999; Mensah, 2003; Héritier, 2013).

Methods

Between 2013 and 2016, I conducted 30 in-depth interviews with women living with HIV in the French-speaking part of Switzerland. All were diagnosed HIV-positive prior to 2000. This time frame was set to study their life course trajectories in terms of their experiences with the virus and their medical treatment and management. The choice to conduct a study with women living with HIV who are not sex workers, drug users or from a country with high HIV prevalence is to address a gap in the history of HIV/AIDS. The participants in this study represent a minority in Switzerland that is unstudied and particularly invisible (Fargnoli, 2021).[2]

Seventeen participants were recruited through the medical community, nine through specialised associations, two via social and professional networks and two with snowball sampling (where one participant recruits another participant). Potential participants were given a letter that outlined the research objectives and explained how data would be used. All participants signed an informed consent document before the interviews began. With the permission of participants, interviews were audio-recorded and transcribed verbatim.

Two interviews were carried out with each participant. The interview guide covered two main topics: the period of HIV-positive diagnosis, including participants' reactions to their test results and who they informed about their diagnosis; and the daily management of HIV, including the evolution of their networks (social, medical, professional), their medical treatment(s) and relationships with doctors and healthcare givers, and the impact of HIV on their sexual lives.

Interview transcripts were coded using qualitative analysis software (ATLAS.ti). The coding process was conducted in two steps: the interview guide topics provided initial codes; and some inductive codes (such as 'sexual

---

[2] Though not reported on in this chapter, I also conducted ten semi-structured interviews with HIV/AIDS experts, including doctors, nurses, association members and one legal expert. Some of these individuals were gatekeepers for recruiting other participants.

violence' and 'lack of recognition') were created from the data collected. Thematic analysis was adopted (Braun and Clarke, 2006). The analysis of participants' first interviews identified central topics, which were then incorporated into second interviews. During the final stage of the analysis, the main concepts that emerged from the data were 'identity', 'undetectable' and 'invisibility'. These constituted the three main dimensions used in describing: how they became HIV-positive, in the sense of acquiring a new identity (subjective dimension); how they became undetectable, referring to the medical aspect of living and ageing with HIV (biological dimension); and how they became invisible, tackling the issue of stigmatisation and discrimination (social dimension).

The project protocol was approved by two cantonal (that is, state-level) ethical committees. This granted me ethical clearance to recruit participants in the cantons of Geneva and Vaud.

Participant characteristics

Participants' ages at their first interview ranged from 34 to 69 years. They were mainly White and Swiss, living in Switzerland and in France (Grand Geneva). Of the non-Swiss participants, five were from other European countries. Half of the participants were employed (either full time or part time), one was self-employed and nine women were living on disability insurance. All participants identified as heterosexual. Most (19 women) were in heterosexual relationships. Of the 11 single women, two were widows.

Of the 30 participants, 23 had been diagnosed before the introduction of highly active antiretroviral therapies in 1996 in Switzerland. At the time of their HIV test, they were between 19 and 54 years of age. The majority (26 women) were mostly infected in a monogamous heterosexual relationship. Twelve women had given birth after their HIV infection. All these children were born HIV-negative. Twenty-five of the women adhered to an ART regimen.

Although participants had heterogeneous sociocultural profiles, with different levels of education, professional and family status, they did have one thing in common: none had been concerned about HIV/AIDS before their diagnosis, since they did not engage in 'risky behaviours' or belong to key risk populations as defined by the official authorities, such as the World Health Organization, UNAIDS and the FOPH in Switzerland.

In Switzerland, the prevalence of HIV is higher in women between the ages of 35 and 54 than for younger women (FOPH, 2020). Only three of those interviewed had been diagnosed with HIV in their fifties. At the time of their first interviews, 21 were over 50 years of age, and 6 were over 60 years old.

Experiences of women living and ageing with HIV

The experiences of women living and ageing with HIV, presented here, focus on: the impact of HIV on their sexual lives; the corporal HIV experience; and the aspiration to a return to 'normality' through motherhood and relationships.

Impact of HIV on participants' sexual lives

While most of the women interviewed insisted that HIV infection did not prevent them from having fulfilling sexual lives, some reported that they had experienced periods of sexual abstinence immediately after receiving their HIV-positive diagnoses. Many described a "break" or a "blockage" that lasted a couple of months or years: Adèle[3] (52 years old) said, "It took me nine months to be able to make love again", and Charlotte (55 years old) said, "I did a six-year break without having sex." One interviewee, aged 31 at the time of her HIV-positive diagnosis, had not had sex with a man again. Up to the time the research was conducted, she had been abstinent: "I haven't had a single sexual relationship since. It was out of the question. It was clear to me, never again!" (Sybille, 69 years old).

For the interviewees who were not in a relationship, the experiences of intimate discrimination and their ageing bodies have led them to stay single. They frequently explained their sexual inactivity by saying they were not interested any more. This 'sexual retreat' affected eight women at the time of first interview.

For the interviewees who were in a relationship, some described leading "normal" sexual lives, meaning that HIV did not represent an obstacle to their sexual activities. However, some faced changes over time. These changes were related to issues concerning their own health but also that of their partners.

'We haven't had sex in a while. He started to have his urinary problems. But it's not taboo and it's not impossible that [sex] could happen again, but for the moment we are not having any!' (Mia, 56 years old)

'Our sex life took a turn for the worse around 1991–92. He didn't want to talk about it. I tried. I wanted to, but he refused and that was it!' (Jade, 69 years old)

For one participant, it was her husband's unwillingness to engage in protected sex that "closed the sexual chapter". Diagnosed when she was 51 years old,

---

[3] Pseudonyms are used to respect participants' anonymity. The age given relates to the first meeting with the participant.

she made it a condition to her husband, who was HIV-negative, that they would only have sex if condoms were used. She explained that men of her generation (born in the 1940s) used condoms only with sex workers and that her husband justified his unwillingness to have sex with her in that context: "We didn't have sex any more. People of my generation and for men of my generation, condoms are not for decent people like us! He prefers not having sex over having sex with a condom!" (Beatrice, 69 years old).

As highlighted by feminists, the (hetero)patriarchal system ideology constructs women in two divergent roles: mother and whore (Pheterson, 1993; Wilton, 1997). These roles oppose a 'clean' and 'safe' family sexuality with a 'dirty' and 'dangerous' commercial sexuality. It is on the latter construct that women's responsibility to prevent sexually transmitted diseases have been built (Wilton, 1997).

The same sort of sexual abstinence imposed by Beatrice's husband was experienced by other interviewees. One explained that, at the age of 50 and over, heterosexual men do not know how to use condoms or "are very reluctant to use them". 'Sexual retirement' in this context has been imposed by participants' partners. As has been emphasised in the literature, social policy and prevention forgot to target 'older' individuals who are not socialised to 'safe sex', resulting in sex without condoms. Those individuals are, therefore, exposed to higher risk of contracting sexually transmitted diseases (Lusti-Narasimhan and Beard, 2013; Banens et al, 2015).

Some women talked about a sexual disinvestment that had developed over time and which was linked to change in their social status rather than their biological status. For example, from some participants' perspectives, becoming a grandmother appears incompatible with an active sexual life. As previously mentioned, ageing women's bodies and their social status, including gender norms, are embedded in the idea of the biological clock (Shorter, 1984; Wilton, 1997; Ruault, 2015).

Rose, aged 69 years, diagnosed HIV-positive at 54, explained the 'death' of her libido as a consequence of long-term medical treatments rather than part of the ageing process: "As far as sex is concerned, I don't have any libido at all. The treatment really cuts everything off!" For most interviewees, it was difficult to identify whether HIV has had an impact on their ageing or their ageing has had an impact on their illness. A common sentiment was that with or without HIV, you get older! However, the burden of the years lived with the virus appeared heavier for women who have lived with HIV and have been under medical treatment for many years. Some even expressed a feeling of early ageing (Deeks, 2009; Levett et al, 2014) due to HIV. Roxane (53 years old) said:

'I don't know if it's the age or the medication, but it takes me longer to do things [than] before. I feel an excessive fatigue, which is not normal. I'm convinced that when you take ART, you get older and you age faster. I can feel it. I see it!'

Two women, whose husbands had died from the consequences of AIDS, mentioned that they would never be able, as one put it, to go "to bed with another man".

Finally, some participants, single at the time of the interview, specified that they would prefer to have a relationship based on intimate partnership rather than one based on sex. This stresses the burden of loneliness rather than sexual needs when faced with ageing. Jade (69 years old) said: "I am almost 70 years old. I would be interested in having a male friend-partner to have a male presence and opinion. I have a lot of female friends, but none of them are men." Like Jade, most of the 'older' women (those aged over 60), expressed a desire to engage in interactions of emotional intimacy rather than a penetrative sexuality.

Therefore, the cessation of sexual lives among 'older' women, often presented as a personal choice, might be explained to some extent by the gendered and sexual construction of sexuality. In other words, an internalisation of a 'sexualised age' occurs (Ruault, 2015). This cessation can also be due to male-partner sexual issues and choices.

In the case of HIV, the corporal experience of being HIV-positive should also be considered. It affects women in their intimacy, particularly the perceptions they have about their bodies, but also how others perceive their bodies, as 'safe' or 'dangerous'. Indeed, striking representations of the 'dangerous' and 'dirty' body were frequently provided by participants. This 'dangerousness' is a reminder of the heritage of venereal diseases, in which women were categorised as 'reservoirs' of sexually transmitted infections', a statement found as far back as the 15th century (Wilton, 1997).

The corporal HIV experience

Interviewees commonly used phrases like "infected body", "dangerous body", "sick body", "soiled body", "threatened body", "suspected body" to express their bodies' fight against the virus and experience of subsequent medical treatments. These phrases were also used to refer to others' perceptions of their HIV-infected bodies.

For them, "being undetectable", a reference to having an undetectable HIV viral load, did not necessarily mean being healthy, but rather not representing a risk of HIV transmission any more. Some interpreted this status as no longer being "dangerous" or "monstrous". Here, the women expressed a social condition that affects others – a body previously dangerous had become safe for others – more so than a physiological state. However, for some interviewees, the perception of being "contagious" remained. Fanny

(35 years old) said: "It means that I can't transmit it to someone. I am no longer contagious. Even that would scare me. What does this mean? That I am less dangerous than someone who is HIV-positive and who wouldn't know it?"

Some participants expressed a strong feeling of living with a "dirty body": "From a female point of view, sexually, we feel disgusting, dirty, spoiled!" (Deborah, 62 years old). The infectious nature of HIV remains, in their views, strongly embedded in social norms and a powerful level of rejection by others that has not changed over time. Indeed, they strongly believed that they were still perceived as potentially dangerous to others and to society:

'We are always considered like lepers!' (Ariane, 68 years old)

'Not many people today would drink from my cup, lick my spoon, when we know very well that nobody can get AIDS like that! The fears are just as deep as they were back then. People get along intellectually, but fear is just as deep.' (Adèle, 52 years old)

The perception of the threatening body even led to overprotective measures by male partners, such as wearing two condoms or refusing to kiss their partners, giving the impression that for these men the sexual experience was potentially "toxic". This reinforced the image of a dangerous body or one with potential to "kill". As one participant commented: "You are making love with death!"

Therefore, HIV was, and still is, for some interviewees, a major obstacle in their sexual relationships, as the issue of transmission is still unsolved despite medically successful reduction of viral load. Indeed, despite knowing they were not at risk of transmitting HIV (having undetectable viremia), in practice the fear of HIV transmission remained an unacceptable risk for some participants. Tina (52 years old) said: "I am still reluctant to have unprotected sex even if I have a steady partner. I'm never 100 per cent ok. To say we can have sex without a condom, there is always a little doubt about not infecting someone."

In addition, doubts about potential transmission also arose when the HIV-negative partner had weakened immune status: "He was tired, he had a cold. During this period, he said: 'Do you mind if we put condoms back on for two or three months because I don't feel well, I'm tired?'" (Valentine, 44 years old). This comment, along with similar testimonies by other interviewees, illustrates an inability to transform the representation of an HIV-infected body as one that is dangerous and capable of infecting and transmitting 'death' to one that is harmless and treated. According to various authors, the risk of transmission has always significantly altered the sexual and emotional lives of people living with HIV, both before and after ART (Pierret, 2006; Pezeril, 2012).

Negative, violent reactions from sexual partners in so-called 'recreational' sexual settings are common and a direct result of the 'HIV dangerous body'. These experiences have left some participants without sexual and emotional relationships over long periods. Indeed, many reported instances of potential sexual partners leaving, or as one put it, "running away". This reaction confirmed for some that they were still perceived as a 'vessel' of disease. Four participants said they explicitly abandoned their love and sexual lives because of the virus. This sexual abstinence may have been a strategy for avoiding disclosure of HIV status.

Some participants in a stable relationship expressed feelings of "gratitude" and "recognition" towards their "healthy" partners, who they considered "heroes" in reference to their ability to overcome the danger of HIV. In other words, they thought highly of their partners because of their acceptance of the risk of being infected, even where participants had had an undetectable viremia for years. Coralie (41 years old) said: "People who dare to face it are heroes. It's the way I look at myself. I don't deserve it. Whoever dares to [have sex] with me is a hero!"

As Lagrave (2011) highlights, 'the gaze of others constructs old age, but the absence of a desiring gaze puts an end to any desire' (p 2). If some participants still felt sexually desired by their partners, others were still fighting with their undesirable body. This was especially the case for those affected by lipodystrophy. The 'lipodystrophied body' reveals the corporality of ART, not only in a purely aesthetic dimension but also in relation to femininity. Some interviewees claimed that due to lipodystrophy, they no longer felt, as one put it, "like a woman". For them, this meant appearing healthy and beautiful, two social components of Western (hetero)femininity (Théry, 1999).

'Lipodystrophy! You may be 70 years old, but you are still a woman. To say that you are no longer desirable! All this fat that comes here [in the abdominal region]. I don't have any flesh on my thighs. I don't have anything here [cheeks].' (Beatrice, 69 years old)

'The physical image disturbs me. I am ashamed of the fat in the belly and these holes on my cheeks bother me. My face doesn't look healthy. I have the impression that my body is marked by the illness. I am not a woman! I don't feel like a woman!' (Jessica, 47 years old)

Lipodystrophy represents the trace of the infection on participants' bodies and is the physical manifestation of the stigma of HIV. In other words, the 'treated body' (Pierret, 2006) is exposed publicly. This seal of difference through lipodystrophy affected not only their relationships with themselves

("I am no longer a woman"), but also their relationships with others in their intimacy.

'Older' women have to face other body transformations, such as menopause, a stage in their biological clock perceived as a 'normal' end to their sexuality (Ruault, 2015). As one woman said: "It [sexuality] goes with the age. For me, it's not an issue because I'm going through menopause. In life there is a time for everything" (Deborah, 62 years old).

Aspirations to return to 'normality'

In the interviewees' journeys with HIV, experiences such as meeting a partner or the birth of a child blurred the negative feelings they had about themselves with HIV. For many of them, that these things happened even after their HIV-positive diagnosis represented a victory and a sort of revenge against their HIV infection.

Often, meeting a partner after an HIV-positive diagnosis allowed the women living with HIV to feel like "a normal woman" – meaning a woman without HIV – again. Most of the interviewees noted that being married had helped them to overcome the hardship of HIV, as this enabled them to play social roles that are acceptable in heteropatriarchal societies: being a wife and a mother. It was even important to some participants that their infection had taken place when they were in a loving relationship, as opposed to the infection being the result of a fleeting encounter.

The strong impact of childbirth on the experience of women living with HIV could be explained by the strong social injunction to procreate, which weighs more heavily on women than on men. As argued by Delphy (2003), 'for a woman, the status of mother is a determining factor in social status and respect by those around her' (p 57). The women who had chosen not to have a child due to their HIV status expressed an ongoing suffering that was still present at the time of interview. They blamed the virus for having deprived them of the experience of motherhood. Of the 30 participants, 4 had ruled out having a child due to HIV. This was the case for Jessica, who learned her HIV-positive status in 1991 while having a routine check-up in early pregnancy. On receiving her HIV-positive diagnosis, she immediately terminated the pregnancy. A few participants would have liked to expand their families by having more children, but they feared the risk of vertical transmission, even if they had an undetectable viremia. Denying motherhood shows how the female body is affected by HIV, with the body seen not only as fertile (able to give life) but also as unwelcoming (Théry, 1999; Héritier, 2013). However, some women did not mourn motherhood, since they had not planned on having a child.

The desire for normality through having a partner and the fear of being alone, of never meeting someone who might accept their condition, forced some interviewees to stay in unfulfilling relationships. Some recounted experiences of partners who would not commit to long-term relationships or who refused to become a parent with an HIV-positive woman. Tina (52 years old) said: "He called me a cunt! It was just fuck you once and goodbye! It's always the same thing. They don't want to get involved. It hurts! It's not something that's easy to live with!" This narrative suggests that the most damaging consequences of being a woman living with HIV appear in the individual's intimate and sexual life. Even for those who have been undetectable for a long time and may have put their HIV-positive status to the back of their minds, events related to emotional and sexual relationships are inevitable reminders.

Despite time having passed since their HIV-positive diagnosis, the reference to not being "a normal woman", a 'woman like any other' (Théry, 1999, p. 113), was often repeated by participants, indicating that this feeling had not changed over the years. This expression of lacking normality due to HIV also referred to lack of interest by others towards them: "We will never be [normal] and live a normal life! Who cares about us? Who cares about an HIV-positive woman in 2014? Who can still be interested in me? It's still shameful!" (Adèle, 52 years old).

Lack of normality was also reinforced by the transgression of traditional social norms as a result of having an HIV-positive status. Therefore, though some men 'normalised' the women's HIV, others damaged the women's self-esteem and body image, and even their overall self-worth. These social sanctions experienced in the most intimate interactions resulted in a sexual death for some women, not linked with their age.

Limitations and implications

One limitation of the study is the potential for recruitment bias, since participants were mainly recruited by healthcare practitioners (n = 17). I do not know whether the doctors and nurses proposed the study to all eligible patients or asked specific women to participate. Another limitation concerns the scope of the study. Interviews with participants' partners were planned initially, but these were abandoned due to time pressure and limited access to the field. These interviews would have aimed to identify the consequences of HIV for the couples' sexual and romantic lives from the perspective of seronegative males.

The findings of this qualitative study offer some insights and lay groundwork for further research. For the care of people living with HIV, whether it be at the level of social health policy or support from medical establishments or associations, it is necessary to take account of the diversity of experiences, regardless of individuals' belonging, or not, to a key population. One of the reasons given by participants for taking part in this study was to prove that HIV concerns everyone – a message they would like to see relayed more in the media by associations and doctors, and in prevention messages, from which they often feel excluded. In other words, as long as the issue of HIV/AIDS is perceived as affecting only certain target groups, it will be difficult for other people to connect with it. Furthermore, understanding the views of women living with HIV, especially when these views are not in line with dominant definitions or mainstream social norms, could lead to policies that better encapsulate and consider their needs and experiences.

The absence in the official HIV/AIDS history of women living with HIV and, in addition, the absence of studies on the sexual lives of 'older' people reveal a need to study and make visible different experiences. This chapter covers some aspects of what it means to live and to age with HIV for women who are outside of the mainstream representations of HIV/AIDS, and the impact of HIV on their sexual lives. In further research to understand the impact of ageing with HIV and sexuality in later life, specificities of women need to be considered, as ageing does not affect women and men in the same way. Sexuality of 'older' women, with or without HIV, will remain overlooked if the 'fertility frame' persists, shaped by medical heteronormativity and traditional, ageist stereotypes. In this context, 'older' women's sexual needs, desires and erotism will likely remain overshadowed and taboo. Therefore, in the field of HIV, an age-inclusive approach with a gender lens must emerge to give attention to women's specificities and experiences, especially for those who have been excluded from existing social and medical categorisations.

Conclusion

The sexual lives of women ageing with HIV are affected to different degrees. Biologically, long-term medical treatments and the ageing body, linked to menopause, can result in lack of libido and cessation of sexual activities. Socially, women's status is linked with normative life events, such as becoming a mother, that can also impact their sexual lives. In their interactions with partners, experiencing successive failed relationships or having the feeling of not being desirable any more can lead to sexual retirement. Women ageing with HIV therefore face age discrimination, similar to all women, but with the addition of the corporal experience of HIV and discrimination related to that. Indeed, some participants pointed out that the construction of AIDS as a 'dangerous illness' in the 1980s still allows for feelings of hostility and distrust towards people living with HIV but also among people living with HIV. The treated body as non-infectious does not convince everyone. Living with HIV, in this case, means living with the indelible imprint of the history of a threatening epidemic.

HIV infection transgresses and undermines gender role assignments. A mother gives life, not death; a wife preserves and cares for her family's health and does not endanger it (Héritier, 2013). These assignments remained well anchored in the participants' aspirations, and they are also relayed in social and medical interactions. In this study, HIV/AIDS was referred to as the "disease of love", but also the "disease of lack of love". If it was in a loving relationship that the majority of the women interviewed were infected and betrayed, it was also in a loving relationship that they managed to rebuild themselves and reconstruct their lives with HIV. Indeed, this study shows that women living with HIV aspired to achieve typical feminine trajectories, underscoring how a 'successful life' is expressed through strong, long-term relationships and normative family ideals, such as mothering, independent of age. Therefore, the social dimension and consequences of HIV have to be taken into account as the burden of the virus is particularly felt in its relational dimension, making it not only a biological disease but also a disease of relationships.

References

Bajos, N. and Bozon, M. (2008) 'Transformation des comportements, immobilité des représentations', *Informations sociales*, 144: 22–33.

Banens, M., Mendes-Leite, R., Talpin, J.-M. and Cuvillier, B. (2015) *Vieillir avec le VIH: Les séniors séropositifs à Lyon et dans la Vallée du Rhone*, Lyon: Centre Max Weber – CNRS, Université Lumière Lyon 2, Available from: https://halshs.archives-ouvertes.fr/halshs-01247694

Banke-Thomas, A., Olorunsaiye, C.Z. and Yaya, S. (2020) '"Leaving no one behind" also includes taking the elderly along concerning their sexual and reproductive health and rights: a new focus for reproductive health', *Reproductive Health* [online], 17(1): 101. https://doi.org/10.1186/s12978-020-00944-5

Bernard, C., Balestre, E., Coffie, P.A., Eholie, S.P., Messou, E., Kwaghe, V., Okwara, B., Sawadogo, A., Abo, Y., Dabis, F. and de Rekeneire, N. (2018) 'Aging with HIV: what effect on mortality and loss to follow-up in the course of antiretroviral therapy? The IeDEA West Africa Cohort Collaboration', *HIV/AIDS – Research and Palliative Care*, 10: 239–52.

Blanco, J.R., Caro, A.M., Pérez-Cachafeiro, S., Gutiérrez, F., Iribarren, J.A., González-García, J., Ferrando-Martínez, S., Navarro, G. and Moreno, S. (2010) 'HIV infection and aging', *AIDS Reviews*, 12(4): 218–30.

Braun, V. and Clarke, V. (2006) 'Using thematic analysis in psychology', *Qualitative Research in Psychology*, 3(2): 77–101.

Brenot, P. and Wunsch, S. (2016) 'Les attentes sexuelles des femmes face aux attentes de leur partenaire', *Sexologies*, 25(1): 31–4.

Campbell, C.A. (1995) 'Male gender roles and sexuality: implications for women's AIDS risk and prevention', *Social Science & Medicine*, 41(2): 197–210.

Corea, G. (1993) *The Invisible Epidemic: The Story of Women and AIDS*, New York: Harper Perennial.

Deeks, S.G. (2009) 'Immune dysfunction, inflammation, and accelerated aging in patients on antiretroviral therapy', *Topics in HIV Medicine*, 17(4): 118–23.

Delphy, C. (2003) 'Par où attaquer le "partage inégal" du "travail ménager"?', *Nouvelles Questions Féministes*, 22(3): 47–71.

Dorlin, E. (2005) 'Sexe, genre et intersexualité: la crise comme régime théorique', *Raisons politiques*, 2(18): 117–37.

Fargnoli, V. (2021) *Invihsibles: trajectoires de femmes séropositives*, Lausanne: Editions Antipodes.

FOPH (Federal Office of Public Health, Switzerland) (2018a) "Groupes à risque d'exposition élevé (axe 2)" [online], Available from: https://www.bag.admin.ch/bag/fr/home/strategie-und-politik/nationale-gesundheitsstrategien/nationales-programm-hiv-und-andere-sexuell-uebertragbare-infektionen/zielgruppe-mit-erhoehtem-expositionsrisiko-achse2.html

FOPH (Federal Office of Public Health, Switzerland) (2018b) *Statistiques et analyses concernant VIH/IST 2017. VIH, syphilis, gonorrhée et chlamydiose en Suisse en 2017: survol épidémiologique*, Berne: Office fédéral de la santé publique, Available from: https://www.bag.admin.ch/bag/fr/home/zahlen-und-statistiken/zahlen-zu-infektionskrankheiten/hiv-sti-statistiken-analysen-trends.html

FOPH (Federal Office of Public Health, Switzerland) (2020) *Statistiques et analyses concernant VIH/IST 2019. VIH, syphilis, gonorrhée et chlamydiose en Suisse 2019: survol épidémiologique*, Berne: Office fédéral de la santé publique, Available from: https://www.bag.admin.ch/bag/fr/home/zahlen-und-statistiken/zahlen-zu-infektionskrankheiten/hiv-sti-statistiken-analysen-trends.html

Hasse, B., Ledergerber, B., Furrer, H., Battegay, M., Hirschel, B., Cavassini, M., Bertisch, B., Bernasconi, E., Weber, R. and Swiss HIV Cohort Study (2011) 'Morbidity and aging in HIV-infected persons: the Swiss HIV cohort study', *Clinical Infectious Diseases*, 53(11): 1130–9.

Héritier, F. (2013) *Sida, un défi anthropologique*, Paris: Les Belles Lettres.

High, K.P., Brennan-Ing, M., Clifford, D.B., Cohen, M.H., Currier, J., Deeks, S.G., Effros, R.B., Gebo, K., Goronzy, J.J., Justice, A.C., Landay, A., Levin, J., Miotti, P.G., Munk, R.J., Nass, H., Rinaldo, C.R., Shlipak, M.G., Tracy, R., Valcour, V., Vance, D.E., Walston, J.D. and Volberding, P. (2012) 'HIV and aging: state of knowledge and areas of critical need for research. A report to the NIH Office of AIDS Research by the HIV and Aging Working Group', *Journal of Acquired Immune Deficiency Syndrome*, 60(Suppl 1): S1–S18.

Kearney, F., Moore, A.R., Donegan, C.F. and Lambert, J. (2010) 'The ageing of HIV: implications for geriatric medicine', *Age and Ageing*, 39(5): 536–41.

Kergoat, D. (2005) 'Rapports sociaux et division du travail entre les sexes', in M. Maruani (ed) *Femmes, genre et sociétés*, Paris: La Découverte, pp 94–101.

Lagrave, R.-M. (2011) 'L'impensé de la vieillesse: la sexualité', *Genre, sexualité & société* [online], 6, Available from: http://journals.openedition.org/gss/2154

Latham, B.C., Sowell, R.L. and Phillips, K.D. (2001) 'Family functioning and motivation for childbearing among HIV-infected women at increased risk for pregnancy', *Journal of Family Nursing*, 7(4): 345–70.

Levett, T., Wright, J. and Fisher, M. (2014) 'HIV and ageing: what the geriatrician needs to know', *Reviews in Clinical Gerontology*, 24(1): 10–24.

Lusti-Narasimhan, M. and Beard, J.R. (2013) 'Sexual health in older women', *Bulletin of the World Health Organization*, 91(9): 707–9.

McIntosh, R.C. and Rosselli, M. (2012) 'Stress and coping in women living with HIV: a meta-analytic review', *AIDS and Behavior*, 16(8): 2144–59.

Mensah, M. (2003) *Ni vues ni connues*, Montréal: Les Éditions du Remue-Ménage.

Mottier, V. (2008) *Sexuality: A Very Short Introduction*, Oxford: Oxford University Press.

Pezeril, C. (2012) *Premiers résultats de l'enquête "Les conditions de vie des personnes séropositives en Belgique francophone (Wallonie et Bruxelles)"*, Brussels: Observatoire du sida et des sexualités, Plate-forme Prévention Sida, Available from: https://www.observatoire-sidasexualites.be/wp-content/uploads/publications-et-documents/2012-enquete-conditionsde vie.pdf

Pheterson, G. (1993) 'The whore stigma: female dishonor and male unworthiness', *Social Text*, 37: 39–64.

Pierret, J. (2006) *Vivre avec le VIH: enquête de longue durée auprès des personnes infectées*, Paris: Presses Universitaires de France.

Poglia Mileti, F., Mellini, L., Villani, M., Susltarova, B. and Singy, P. (2014) 'Liens sociaux, secrets et confidences. Le cas des femmes migrantes d'Afrique subsaharienne et séropositives', *Recherches sociologiques et anthropologiques*, 45-2: 167–84.

Rosenbrock, R., Dubois-Arber, F., Moers, M., Pinell, P., Schaeffer, D. and Setbon, M. (2000) 'The normalization of AIDS in Western European countries', *Social Science & Medicine*, 50(11): 1607–29.

Ruault, L. (2015) 'La force de l'âge du sexe faible. Gynécologie médicale et construction d'une vie féminine', *Nouvelles Questions Feministes*, 34(1): 35–50.

Shorter, E. (1984) *Le corps des femmes*, Paris: Seuil.

Théry, I. (1999) '"Une femme comme les autres": séropositivité, sexualité et féminité', in *Séropositivité, vie sexuelle et risque de transmission du VIH*, Paris: Agence Nationale de Recherches sur le Sida, pp 113–36.

Treichler, P.A. (1987) 'AIDS, homophobia and biomedical discourse: an epidemic of signification', *Cultural Studies*, 1(3): 263–305.

Webel, A.R., Cuca, Y., Okonsky, J.G., Asher, A.K., Kaihura, A. and Salata, R.A. (2013) 'The impact of social context on self-management in women living with HIV', *Social Science & Medicine*, 87: 147–54.

Wilton, T. (1997) *Engendering AIDS: Deconstructing Sex, Text and Epidemic*, London: Sage.

World Health Organization (2016) *Stratégie mondiale du secteur de la santé contre le VIH 2016–2021: vers l'élimination du SIDA*, Technical documents, Geneva: World Health Organization, Available from: https://apps.who.int/iris/handle/10665/250576

2

Beyond the biomedical: HIV as a barrier to intimacy for older women living with HIV in the United Kingdom

Jacqui Stevenson

Introduction

'I said I just couldn't [have a relationship], I just, I just don't feel like I could. I'd feel, it's that stigma thing. I'd feel like they would automatically assume that I was a promiscuous woman, and I would just wanna die, so I thought I'd rather do without really.' (Woman living with HIV, aged 70–80, participating in a workshop in London)

HIV has changed. Thanks to extraordinary advances in treatment, people living with HIV who are diagnosed promptly and have access to treatment and care have a near normal life expectancy and can expect the impact of the virus on their daily lives to be limited (May et al, 2014). Consequently, increasing numbers of people are ageing with HIV, leading to new experiences, both positive and negative, around growing older with HIV. Advances in treatment are symbiotically linked with advances in prevention, as it is now established that people on effective HIV treatment with undetectable viral loads cannot transmit the virus, a principle known as undetectable = untransmittable, or U=U (UNAIDS, 2018).

HIV has not changed. Social attitudes to HIV are not keeping pace with clinical progress (National AIDS Trust and Fast-Track Cities London, 2021), and though many attitudes are more informed and less stigmatising, stigma and discrimination persist and talking about HIV can have negative consequences (Public Health England, 2020). Knowledge of advances in HIV treatment and prevention is limited, particularly in communities where risk of HIV is low and limited priority is given to informing people about HIV (National AIDS Trust and Fast-Track Cities London, 2021).

HIV is complicated. To live with HIV is to live with a long-term condition that is manageable with treatment, and with a diagnosis that may have been delivered with a terminal prognosis. It is an identity and marker of community belonging, and a stigmatised condition that potentially opens up the risk of discrimination, judgment or worse. The quote that opens this chapter is from a woman in her seventies, diagnosed with HIV less than five years before she spoke these words in a workshop conducted for this research.[1] She had not interacted socially with other women living with HIV prior to this workshop. Her words were met with support and with challenge by the others in the room. Some understood or shared her feelings, while others encouraged her to believe that stigma, so often self-imposed, could be overcome and that sex and intimacy could be part of her future.

Women ageing with HIV may experience HIV as a barrier to intimate relationships, sex and intimacy. Drawing on the findings of a qualitative study conducted in London between 2015 and 2019, this chapter explores the views and experiences of women diverse in sexuality, gender identity, ethnicity, length of time living with HIV and age. Through participatory, creative methods, including body mapping workshops and life story interviews, women aged over 50 living with HIV described this status as a potential barrier to sex, intimacy and/or relationships. The author expresses her sincere gratitude to all the women living with HIV who contributed to the research.

Importantly, women living with HIV do not live single-issue lives, and other intersecting factors influence their experiences and views around sex and intimacy. These factors include ageism, sexism, anti-trans discrimination and past experiences of sexual and gender-based violence. Partners' attitudes, wider society and diverse life experiences all influence sex and sexual behaviours in older women living with HIV, indicating the limitations of an increasingly biomedicalised HIV response (Young et al, 2019). For this reason, a feminist participatory approach was adopted in this research. The feminist approach sought to address power dynamics within the study and considered the role and impact of gender in women's experiences. In seeking to explore the experiences of an under-represented, diverse and frequently invisible group, the feminist participatory approach enabled an intersectional outlook that considered women's lives in both breadth and depth. It aimed to avoid the limitations inherent in a biomedicalised approach that views all experiences through the prism of illness and treatment. By involving women living with HIV in each stage of the research, from conceptualisation of research questions to literature review and data analysis, women's voices were centred and shaped the direction, content and findings of the research.

The main research questions explored in this study were: What are the experiences of women ageing with HIV in London? How are these

---

[1] The data presented in this chapter were collected as part of the author's PhD study. An overview of the research and publications from it can be found in Stevenson, 2022 or at: https://sophiaforum.net/wp-content/uploads/2020/09/Im-Still-Here-research-summ ary-Dr-Jacqui-Stevenson.pdf

experiences understood and expressed? A number of sub-questions were also explored, including: How are these experiences mediated by gender, sexuality, ethnicity, migration status and experiences, or other factors? The study was constructed broadly, recognising that the evidence base on women's experiences of ageing with HIV is limited and that existing studies often focus narrowly on HIV, potentially missing the wider intersectional experiences that are integral to the full and rich lives of women growing older with HIV. In the UK context, race, ethnicity and migration are significant intersecting experiences for many women living with HIV, and this study aimed to create space to explore the diversity of individual and collective experience through participatory approaches.

In this chapter, an overview of women, ageing and HIV in the UK context is presented, followed by a consideration of biomedicalisation in the context of HIV and its limitations in capturing the rich and intersecting experiences of those living and ageing with HIV. The methodology and study participants are then described, followed by the findings in relation to sex and intimacy.

Women, ageing and HIV

The research presented in this chapter was conducted in the United Kingdom, where women are a minority among people living with HIV, so their specific needs and experiences are under-researched and under-prioritised (Sophia Forum and Terrence Higgins Trust, 2018). At the time the research was carried out, women made up 29 per cent of people living with HIV in the United Kingdom (Public Health England, 2018). The proportion of the those living with HIV who are of older age is increasing: 39 per cent of people who received HIV care in the United Kingdom in 2017 were aged over 50 (Public Health England, 2018). New diagnoses among older people are increasing: 20 per cent of new diagnoses in 2017 were for people aged over 50, compared with 11 per cent in 2008 (Public Health England, 2018). As the population of people living with HIV ages, so do the medical and social care needs of patient cohorts change, including those associated with ageing.

Women ageing with HIV can expect to experience healthcare needs linked to ageing – those related to increasing comorbidities and health conditions such as cancers, diabetes and frailty – in the same way as women not living with HIV (Oursler et al, 2011; Smit et al, 2015). In addition, they may also experience conditions caused by long-term antiretroviral treatment and/or HIV itself, such as kidney and bone density problems (Gupta et al, 2005). The psychological impact of ageing, mental health conditions and polypharmacy may also affect older women living with HIV (Power et al, 2010; Durvasula, 2014; Winston and Underwood, 2015). Additionally, they may experience social care needs due to mobility or physical health problems, or the impact of dementia or related conditions.

Many of these challenges are familiar to anyone who is ageing, but women living with HIV face additional layers of complication, due to both the HIV-specific health burden and the social and psychological impact of HIV. Social isolation and lack of support may be an issue (Rosenfeld et al, 2015). The experience or expectation of stigma and discrimination may present barriers to seeking or benefiting from care and support (Emlet, 2006). Long-term diagnosed women may struggle to plan for and negotiate an older age they never expected to reach (Power et al, 2010). Recently diagnosed older women may face challenges as they negotiate older age with an unexpected HIV diagnosis (Rosenfeld et al, 2015). Whether HIV is a long-term or recent diagnosis, it influences and alters the experience of ageing (Rosenfeld et al, 2015).

Challenges associated with ageing are compounded by the overall challenges that women living with HIV face. Research in London suggests women living with HIV have three times the rate of poor treatment outcomes compared to gay men, with greater issues with adherence and a greater likelihood of detectable viral load (Burch et al, 2015). The difference in treatment outcomes can be partially attributed to socio-economic factors, including poverty and unstable housing (O'Connell, 2015). It may also speak to the ongoing stigmatisation of HIV in the wider community, which creates barriers for women accessing testing, treatment and care, and limits the sources of specialised support available (Johnson et al, 2015).

Ageing with any chronic condition can bring challenges, such as reducing individual ability to manage health and amplifying the effects of the condition (Giddings et al, 2007; Hewitt-Taylor et al, 2013). The additional burden of stigma can magnify these challenges. Given the complex experience of ageing with HIV, older women living with HIV may find sex, relationships and intimacy challenging. While the study presented in this chapter focused on women's experiences of ageing with HIV broadly, the participatory approach created space for women to share experiences across a range of issues, including sex and relationships.

Biomedicalisation of HIV

Women living with HIV are also living full, varied lives with multiple and overlapping identities, relationships and communities. Ageing well is not just about managing HIV – an undetectable viral load is an inadequate measure for a good or meaningful life. Yet the prevailing narrative around HIV has become increasingly biomedicalised, as advances in HIV in recent years have centred on treatment and its corresponding impact on prevention (Young et al, 2019). Biomedicalisation is not a new phenomenon in the context of HIV, but the scale and breadth of its application across all aspects of life, including ageing, has magnified as treatment has advanced.

Biomedicalisation is defined by the 'extension of medical jurisdiction over health itself' as opposed to just 'illness, disease and injury', leading to a commodification of health and conferring individual ethical obligations to seek, maintain and improve it (Clarke et al, 2003, p 162). This includes an extension of the medical realm to natural processes, such as ageing, which is reconceptualised as something to manage, delay or subvert rather than as an inevitable process. Biomedicalisation reconceptualises health as something to be achieved, with individuals viewed as active partners in the pursuit of good health through their managing treatment, exercising, eating well and so on (Rose, 2001). In the context of HIV in the modern treatment era, compliance with treatment and 'achieving' an undetectable viral load are prioritised and imbued with an ethical imperative while the many other facets of life with HIV, such as relationships or social support, are given less attention.

Biomedical approaches are not sufficient to address the complexity of life and experience. Living well with HIV involves managing not just treatment but also stigma, intimacy, relationships, well-being and many other things. In the context of prevention, a biomedical approach posits U=U as a solution to stigma and discrimination in sex and relationships. But this fails to account for the broader barriers that exist around emotional and psychological well-being and safety, partner attitudes and social and community norms.

Methods

The research was structured in overlapping phases and took a feminist and participatory approach. The methods were: participatory literature review; participatory creative workshops; stakeholder interviews; life story interviews; and a participatory analysis workshop. The data presented in this chapter were collected through the participatory creative workshops and life story interviews, and analysed collaboratively in the participatory analysis workshop.

This study was reviewed and granted ethical approval by the University of Greenwich Research Ethics Committee. The committee approved participant information sheets and informed consent forms as well as data storage and other considerations. All participants provided informed consent to take part in the study.

Three participatory creative workshops were conducted, with 18 women taking part. The workshops included icebreaker and other group activities, facilitated discussion using focus group techniques, and creative exercises. The participatory approach involved women living with HIV in defining the key areas for exploration in the study, shaping the research questions and identifying priorities within and beyond the topic of HIV. This responded to the limitations of a biomedicalised approach by creating space for women, beyond the role of patient and recipient of care, to actively shape the research.

The creative exercise was an adaptation of 'body mapping', a technique developed in South Africa with an HIV support group (Solomon, 2007). Body mapping is a creative tool used, in multi-day workshops, to support participants to engage in feelings and reflections about adapting to living with HIV. For this study, some key elements of body mapping were adapted to a short activity that participants completed individually. Each woman was provided with paper and pens and asked to complete the mapping process independently. The mapping process involved six stages: drawing the body; using symbols and pictures to illustrate where you have come from; using symbols and pictures to describe where you are going; describing your support base; drawing on physical pains and marks; and finally drawing on emotional pains and marks (see an example in Figure 2.1). After moving through the six stages and completing their body maps, each participant narrated their map, without interruption. This narration was included as verbatim data in the analysis. The creative process carved out space for each woman to reflect on her experiences and choose what to share and how to share it, and the individual, uninterrupted narration allowed for these experiences to be shared in a more full and independent way than would be possible with a focus group approach.

The research also included life story interviews with 14 women. This method creates space for a more balanced and wide-ranging research encounter. Interviews opened with the prompt 'where would you like to begin?' Additional prompts were used only when necessary as participants shared their stories. Participants had scope to shape the direction of the interview and determine what to share, and they could ascribe meaning to their stories and experiences.

In the final phase of this research, participatory data analysis was conducted in a workshop with four older women living with HIV. This was based on a participatory analysis process described by a social sector impact organisation, Learning for Action (nd), and adapted to this project. Participants analysed transcript excerpts, developed and grouped codes, and explored meanings and themes from the data.

Participants

Participants in the participatory creative workshops and life story interviews were recruited through social media, newsletters and direct outreach from peer support and third sector organisations who supported the study. In this qualitative study, the number of participants was necessarily small and not intended to be representative, but participants were selected to ensure

Figure 2.1: An example of a body map generated by study participants

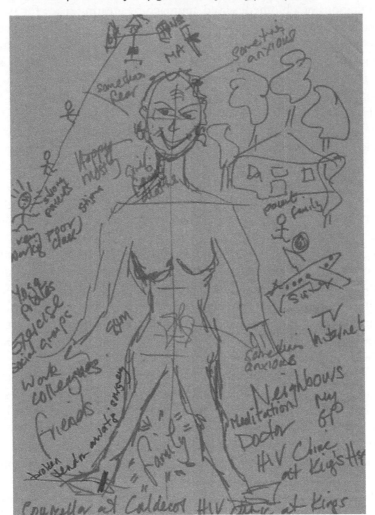

diversity across key identifiers including age, ethnicity and length of diagnosis with HIV.

Two workshops had five participants and one had eight participants. Thirteen of the women were aged 50–59, four were aged 60–69, and one was aged 70–79. Fifteen participants described their ethnicity as Black African, and three as White British; the former migrated to the United Kingdom, while the latter were born in the United Kingdom. Of the 15 who had migrated to the United Kingdom, 12 were born in East and Southern Africa, 1 was born in West and Central Africa, and 2 did not provide this information. Fifteen of the women described themselves as single, one as married and two as widowed. Ten described themselves as having a disability, and five had no disability (of the remaining participants, two did not disclose whether they had a disability and one responded that they do 'sometimes'). The time since diagnosis with HIV varied from seven months to 27 years, with most participants having been diagnosed for 10–15 years.

Of the 14 women who took part in life story interviews, 7 described their ethnicity as Black African, 5 as White British, 1 as White other and 1 as Black British. Nine were migrants to the United Kingdom. Twelve were aged 50–59, and two were aged 60–69. Two identified as bisexual, and one identified as trans. Length of time diagnosed with HIV varied: less than five years for one woman, five to ten years for three women, and over ten years for ten women. Five described themselves as currently in a relationship, seven as single, one as separated and one as divorced.

Participatory analysis

All data from workshops and life story interviews were fully transcribed and anonymised, with pseudonyms used in place of real names. Thematic analysis was conducted through a process of organising the data, coding, condensing codes to generate themes and representing the data (Creswell and Poth, 2017). After developing a draft analytical framework of themes and categories, a participatory analysis workshop was conducted to involve older women living with HIV in interpretation of the data. Four women participated in the workshop, and they each consented to being identified in all outputs associated with the study, to acknowledge their invaluable contribution. The women were: Angelina Namiba, advocate, facilitator and trainer for women living with HIV; Memory Sachikonye, coordinator of UK Community Advisory Board (UK-CAB) and co-chair of Sophia Forum; Silvia Petretti, deputy CEO of Positively UK and advocate; and Jane Shepherd, advocate and UK-CAB committee member. All were women living with HIV, aged over 50, with professional or voluntary experience in supporting, working with or representing women living with HIV, which enabled them to bring a broad and informed perspective to the analysis.

Prior to the workshop, each participant received by email an eight-page document that contained: an introduction to the research; a summary of the research design; the purpose of the workshop; research questions; demographics of life story interview participants; and data samples for analysis. The latter were excerpts from six life story interviews, selected for diversity of participant demographics and to reflect the different aspects or topics that came up in the interviews.

Participants were asked to read the document in advance, if possible, and they also had time within the workshop to review it. The agenda involved: individual review of transcripts and open coding; each participant putting forward three codes for the participants to work on; creating groups, adding remaining codes and developing or expanding groups; reviewing remaining transcripts separately and adding any new codes that emerged; and a broad discussion of any gaps. Finally, the draft analytical framework was shared with participants for discussion, in particular to identify any gaps based on their own analysis.

Subsequently, the analytical framework was revised by the author, based on the participatory analysis workshop and further analysis of all the data in the study. The final framework was used to code the data using NVivo 11 software. Of the many benefits of the participatory analysis workshop was the identification of gaps in both women's stories and the preliminary analysis. One such gap was the issue of sex and intimacy.

Sex and intimacy

Women participating in this study talked openly about many aspects of their lives, from HIV diagnosis to experiences of bereavement, violence, ill health and motherhood. However, as identified by participants in the analysis workshop, sex was rarely mentioned explicitly, and for many women, as in the quote that opened this chapter, it was described as something that was out of reach or no longer desired. Sex was seldom part of women's lives or future imaginings, indicating that advances in HIV prevention have not necessarily opened up opportunities for women ageing with HIV. While women were often familiar with the science of U=U, this was not sufficient to change their experiences or their expectations around sex and sexual opportunity. Transmission of HIV was not the main barrier or concern described by the women; rather it was stigmatising, hurtful, judgmental or even violent reactions from partners. For some women, intimacy was necessarily associated with sharing their HIV status with potential partners, which was difficult and risk laden. Consequently, for many women, HIV was a barrier to sex and intimate relationships. Women described a hard choice between sharing their HIV status in order to achieve intimacy, risking judgment and negative consequences, or keeping their status hidden and, as they understood it, preventing true intimacy by maintaining this secrecy.

The life story interview prompts did not ask directly about sex, but in some interviews the prompt 'what does intimacy mean to you?' was used. In response, most women talked about emotional support, feeling close to others and connection. While concerns about transmission of HIV were discussed, often that was not the main consideration. This is important not just because it indicates that sex seemed not to feature in women's current lives or future plans, but also because it helps in understanding how and why HIV is a barrier to relationships. Since, for most women, the concern was not about transmission, scientific advances around U=U were not enough to address the barriers these women were experiencing. Indeed, for both bisexual women interviewed, the possibility of being with a woman, with virtually zero transmission risk, did not open up intimacy or partnerships.

Yvette, a 58-year-old Black African woman, diagnosed for 16 years, described trust and support as more important than sex, which felt out of reach for her as she struggled to overcome difficult experiences including rape, abusive relationships, homelessness and immigration challenges. For her, the risks of talking about HIV with a partner and of opening up to intimacy felt too great to overcome.

'I don't even think about it actually. No. It's gone. I think, to me, its trust. I don't trust. And I, it's not just about sex, I don't … my feelings as well. I don't like people playing with my feelings, so I just cut it off. I'm happy, my friends make me happy, I laugh, I do things. The only thing I don't do is sex, and I'm not missing it.' (Yvette)

Tindo, aged 54 and Black African, had faced significant loss and trauma, including the death of her husband, being raped and migrating to a new country with no social support network. Like Yvette, she was concerned with the risks involved in developing intimate relationships. Though she still hoped it was a possibility, she described a desire for formal support to navigate this safely.

'If I could I don't mind. I need a friend. But I'm a very, I'm so scared through what I've gone through. I haven't had a boyfriend since I came in this country, because of the trauma I have … But if it is through professional people who can introduce us, I would feel comfortable. But on my own to meet someone and think I can talk to this person and, I'm so scared. Very scared. But I would love to be with someone. I would love to be with someone who would be there for me if I'm ill. And I, the same as him as well, just to look after each other at our age. Because my kids, they're grown-ups, they've got their lives. They can't be there for me 24/7. So it's time for me to be with someone. A responsible person, because I know I'm a responsible woman as well. But through people who will be checking on us to see if everything is ok. Because this is a foreign country. It's different from back home where you are introduced to a family member where you know the family. That's why I'm so scared.' (Tindo)

For Patricia, a 50-year-old Black African woman, the barriers to sex and relationships posed by HIV were the practical challenges of managing treatment, side effects and pain.

'I used to, once upon a time I had intimacy but, you know, when your life is taken over by, you're taking medication, you're having side effects, you're ... I think my priority now is just staying well, rather than looking for a relationship. So, for me, intimacy's when you're, you're in it because it's good for you, because it helps you. I mean, you give and you take, you know, two-way system, and, and you're not complicating it with your own situation, which I feel, you know, I feel I have baggage at the moment ... my priorities have switched, with just bearing with the pain.' (Patricia)

HIV was not a barrier to sex and relationships for all the women who took part in this research, though it did affect relationships in different ways. Alice, a 68-year-old White British woman feared that her activism and decision to be public about her HIV status would prevent her from forming sexual relationships but, in practice, found that some partners did not find HIV to be an issue. Michelle, aged 50 and diagnosed for 16 years, also had partners since her diagnosis and found that they reacted well to learning her status, although HIV had caused other issues related to prevention, as one partner had to take post-exposure prophylaxis after a condom failed and another partner found frequent HIV testing difficult.

Secrets and intimacy

For the women in this study, decisions around whether, when and how to talk about HIV presented an ongoing challenge in relationships of all kinds: intimate relationships, family relationships and friendships. The act of keeping their HIV status a secret was a burden not just emotionally and psychologically but also in practical terms when accessing emotional and social support from others, as women described feeling unable to ask for help without being able to explain why they needed it. Throughout this study, women treated telling a partner about their HIV status as inevitable and necessary, sometimes in relation to HIV transmission and prevention, but also for intimacy and support. Even where the risks of transmission were zero, HIV would still need to be discussed.

In the context of increasing biomedicalisation of the HIV response, risk around discussing HIV can be reduced to a focus on the risk of HIV transmission alone, such that U=U becomes a panacea for all potential harms associated with the act of revealing one's HIV status. For example, the Terrence Higgins Trust, a UK charity focused on HIV and sexual health, includes the following on the web page for its Can't Pass It On campaign:

We're telling everyone: someone living with HIV and on effective treatment can't pass it on.

It's one of the most positive messages someone living with HIV can hear. It reduces the stigma around HIV and provides motivation to stay on treatment to keep both themselves and their sexual partners healthy.

If everyone knew this simple and powerful message, we could bring an end to stigma around HIV. Not only that, but we could stop HIV transmissions altogether. (Terrence Higgins Trust, nd)

As a campaign message, this inevitably veers into rhetoric, but it is instructive to consider the premise explicit in this text: stigma is a function of risk or fear of transmission, so successful preventive interventions can end stigma. That is not the story of stigma told by women in this study, who instead described a multifaceted, ongoing conception of stigma, partly internalised and partly externally enacted, that intersected with other forms of discrimination, including sexism, ageism, racism, anti-migrant discrimination and anti-trans discrimination. Just as women do not lead single-issue lives, stigma is not the product of a single cause, so while women in this study were often very well informed about HIV prevention, including U=U and other biomedical prevention tools, this alone was not sufficient to reduce fears of stigma and speaking about HIV with potential partners. Despite biomedical advances, the experience of HIV remained a significant part of these women's lives, posing the risk of rejection when it is revealed to a potential partner but also creating a barrier to true intimacy when it is kept secret. Women often felt HIV was a part of them, of their experiences and their needs for support, and in keeping it hidden, the potential for intimate partnership is lessened. As Patricia noted, contrasting her feelings of safety in forming relationships and community with other people living with HIV, compared to those not living with HIV (who she described broadly as the "normal" community):

'You can build your own community, create your own community, other than the normal communities that are supposed to be there. Especially the normal community, sometimes if they don't know, if you're living with a, a secret disease that you don't wanna share with people, it then becomes difficult to explain yourself.' (Patricia)

HIV is more than a virus, and biomedical solutions can only address biomedical challenges. Talking about HIV was a barrier to sex and relationships because of its implications for intimacy and support, and the risk of negative responses, and these issues are not addressed by prevention of transmission, however effective it may be.

Moreover, for study participants, sharing their HIV status and inviting someone into the intimacy of understanding and supporting their full lives, including HIV, was not a one-off act of 'disclosure', prepared for and supported by educating their partner about HIV prevention and the effectiveness of biomedical interventions. Indeed, participants in the analysis workshop discussed the term 'disclosure' and agreed that its negative, legalistic connotations and the implication that this involves a single act render it inappropriate for conversations about health and identity. They preferred to think of 'talking about HIV', and this as a continuum rather than a one-off act.

Talking about HIV as a continuum involves revealing some information at one time, more at another time, or some details with some people and not with others. Not a 'big reveal', but instead a measured, careful, gradual sharing of personal information and a building of intimacy. This continuum of sharing and discussing the experience of HIV was evident in the narratives of many women in this study. While some had not shared their HIV status at all outside of clinics and support groups, others talked very openly about their HIV, even in national media. But even where this openness was evident, individuals still had limits on when and with whom HIV should be discussed, and challenges in considering why and how to do so. Even those women who were happy to speak about HIV did so with restrictions. Yvette described being happy to speak openly but not to discuss how she acquired HIV, as she felt this supports a culture of blame and obscures the fact that anyone can acquire HIV.

Decisions around talking about HIV often involved consideration of risks and benefits, weighing up whether it would be worthwhile. In the context of intimate partnerships, the risk was, for some women, greater than the potential benefits, leading them to leave the prospect of sex and relationships behind. For others, the risk had been worth taking, often thanks to feeling supported and informed to discuss HIV openly. Importantly, other intersecting experiences and identifiers impacted on the assessment of risk and benefit as women managed the complexity of their lives with and beyond HIV.

Intersectional experiences

In addition to age and HIV status, when recruited to the workshops or life story interviews, women were asked about a range of other characteristics: ethnicity, length of diagnosis with HIV, migration history, sexuality, relationship status, work status, motherhood and disability. Collecting this demographic data enabled a richer analysis that could consider intersecting experiences. Intersectionality is a critical concept in feminist research, developed by Kimberlé Crenshaw (1989) as an analytical frame to recognise and account for discrimination and marginalisation across multiple axes, such as race, ethnicity, sex, gender identity, class, sexual orientation and age. An intersectional analysis allows for a more complete understanding of the experiences of older women living with HIV, accounting for stigma and discrimination, both feared and experienced, across their multiple and complex identities and experiences. This contrasts with a biomedical approach that centres HIV and accounts for only this single axis of marginalisation and disadvantage.

The women who participated in this study described a range of barriers to sex and intimacy, including but also going far beyond HIV. In some cases, these barriers interlinked with HIV, but in others, HIV was secondary or even absent. For example, menopause and ageing could also be a barrier to intimate partnerships for some women. Women attending one workshop described the menopause as decreasing their interest in sex and making it more difficult to find a relationship due to changes in mood.

'And I, and I get a big problem which I can't explain to anyone. It is like HIV again. I get another HIV, which I am fighting there, the what, menopause. I find it very difficult. I was someone who was attractive, like someone who everyone was going to like, sex. But for me no more. I don't have any feeling in it.' (Workshop participant, Black African woman, aged 50–60, diagnosed for over 25 years)

Women who had children sometimes noted that their focus was on them, leaving little time or energy to seek a relationship with a partner. Angela, a 55-year-old with two teenage children, described feeling ready to explore romantic relationships now her children were older and more independent, and having resolved an abusive situation with a former partner.

'It's only since I've been in my fifties I've started to have relationships with other people. It's just, you know, I wasn't even thinking about it. I just like, I'm just there for the kids, it's, I was just glad not to have war. If I didn't have somebody at war with me, that's fine, I'll just take that, you know. But now I actively think I actually [want to] have attention please, that would be very nice, nice attention.' (Angela)

Similarly, for Patsy, a trans woman living with HIV for 24 years who participated in a life story interview, it was HIV in combination with other factors, in her case being trans and over 50, that meant sex, relationships and intimacy felt inaccessible, as she felt society viewed women like her as unattractive and undesirable. The lack of recognition of the sexual needs and sexual agency of women living with HIV, and the contrast with support available to men, especially gay men, living with HIV, was marked for Patsy, and she highlighted this gap as reinforcing gendered norms around sexual risk and desire.

Limitations and implications

This research aimed to increase understanding of women's experiences of ageing with HIV. This study could have been improved by recruiting more women aged 60 and over, and more women diagnosed recently with HIV; further research including women from each group would be beneficial. Additionally, more focused exploration of women's experiences of sex and intimacy would be valuable. The findings from this study indicate the limitations of a biomedicalised approach to HIV and the social, emotional and psychological implications of ageing with HIV that a biomedical approach cannot address. Social and peer support remain critical in supporting women to age well with HIV, along with but not replaced by HIV treatment.

Conclusion

Women in the participatory analysis workshop noted that sex and relationships were often absent from the stories women shared in this study, and even that the women felt these were no longer part of their lives or futures. This grew from HIV, but also from ageing, menopause, caring responsibilities and other experiences. Fear of talking about HIV was only partly lessened by the emergence of U=U, and fears persisted around stigma and negative reactions. Many women had experiences of rape and other forms of violence that affected their views and priorities around sex and intimacy. As women negotiate older age with HIV, they face many challenges, including ageing, menopause, health concerns, HIV treatment side effects, changing caring responsibilities and relationships with children, bereavement, traumatic experiences (including violence), and intersecting stigma and discrimination.

Within the UK context, the disproportionate burden of HIV among African women and the experiences of racism and a hostile immigration system which many of these women share indicate how essential an intersectional approach is to effectively addressing the needs and priorities of women ageing with HIV. Advances in biomedical HIV prevention hold significant potential for alleviating the risk of HIV transmission during sex, but the barriers to sex and intimacy for older women living with HIV are much more complex and varied. It is critical that support provided to women growing older with HIV in the United Kingdom is intersectional and addresses stigma and discrimination based on age, race, migration status, gender identity and other factors. Historically, the HIV response in the United Kingdom has paid limited attention to gender, a deficit that was identified by some women participating in this study, who described feeling left out of support and left behind in biomedicalised narratives of HIV.

Talking about sex and intimacy may also be a challenge due to gender norms and negative social attitudes around sex for women, and past experiences of violence or abuse, so this research is just a starting point in terms of understanding sex and intimacy for older women living with HIV. An important start is recognising that sex, intimacy, sexual pleasure and even sexual risk are things that women want, enjoy and are entitled to. Equally important is acknowledging that for some women, sex is not a priority, and intimacy is possible and desirable in many different forms. HIV is not just a virus, and intimacy is not just sex. Each are as rich, complex and varied as the lives and experiences of women ageing with HIV.

References

Burch, L., Smith, C., Lampe, F., Phillips, A. and Johnson, M. (2015) 'Is the gender difference in viral load response to ART narrowing over time?', 15th European AIDS Conference, Barcelona, Available from: https://www.natap.org/2015/EACS/EACS_39.htm

Clarke, A.E., Shim, J.K., Mamo, L., Fosket, J.R. and Fishman, J.R. (2003) 'Biomedicalization: technoscientific transformations of health, illness, and U.S. biomedicine', *American Sociological Review*, 68(2): 161–94.

Crenshaw, K. (1989) 'Demarginalizing the intersection of race and sex: a Black feminist critique of antidiscrimination doctrine, feminist theory and antiracist politics', *University of Chicago Legal Forum*, 1989(1): 139–67.

Creswell, J.W. and Poth, C.N. (2017) *Qualitative Inquiry and Research Design (International Student Edition): Choosing among Five Approaches* (4th edn), Thousand Oaks, CA: Sage.

Durvasula, R. (2014) 'HIV/AIDS in older women: unique challenges, unmet needs', *Behavioral Medicine*, 40(3): 85–98.

Emlet, C.A. (2006) '"You're awfully old to have this disease": experiences of stigma and ageism in adults 50 years and older living with HIV/AIDS', *The Gerontologist*, 46(6): 781–90.

Giddings, L., Roy, D. and Predeger, E. (2007) 'Women's experience of ageing with a chronic condition', *Journal of Advanced Nursing*, 58(56): 557–65.

Gupta, S.K., Eustace, J.A., Winston, J.A., Boydstun, I.I., Ahuja, T.S., Rodriguez, R.A., Tashima, K.T., Roland, M., Franceschini, N., Palella, F.J., Lennox, J.L., Klotman, P.E., Nachman, S.A., Hall, S.D. and Szczech, L.A. (2005) 'Guidelines for the management of chronic kidney disease in HIV-infected patients: recommendations of the HIV Medicine Association of the Infectious Diseases Society of America', *Clinical Infectious Diseases*, 40(11): 1559–85.

Hewitt-Taylor, J., Bond, C., Hear, S. and Barker, S. (2013) 'The experiences of older people who live with a long-term condition', *Nursing Older People*, 25(6): 21–5.

Johnson, M., Samarina, A., Xi, H., Valdez Ramalho Madruga, J., Hocqueloux, L., Loutfy, M., Fournelle, M.J., Norton, M., Van Wyk, J., Zachry, W. and Martinez, M. (2015) 'Barriers to access to care reported by women living with HIV across 27 countries', *AIDS Care*, 27(10): 1220–30.

Learning for Action (nd) 'Participatory analysis' [online], Available from: http://learningforaction.com/participatory-analysis/

May, M.T., Gompels, M., Delpech, V., Porter, K., Orkin, C., Kegg, S., Hay, P., Johnson, M., Palfreeman, A., Gilson, R., Chadwick, D., Martin, F., Hill, T., Walsh, J., Post, F., Fisher, M., Ainsworth, J., Jose, S., Leen, C., Nelson, M., Anderson, J. and Sabin, C. (2014) 'Impact on life expectancy of HIV-1 positive individuals of CD4+ cell count and viral load response to antiretroviral therapy', *AIDS*, 28(8): 1193–202.

National AIDS Trust and Fast-Track Cities London (2021) *HIV: Public Knowledge and Attitudes*, London: National AIDS Trust, Available from: https://www.nat.org.uk/sites/default/files/publications/HIV%20 Public%20Knowledge%20and%20Attitudes_0.pdf

O'Connell, R. (2015) 'Do socio-economic factors explain gender differences in virological response to ART in the UK?', 15th European AIDS Conference, Barcelona.

Oursler, K.K., Goulet, J.L., Crystal, S., Justice, A.C., Crothers, K., Butt, A.A., Rodriguez-Barradas, M.C., Favors, K., Leaf, D., Katzel, L.I. and Sorkin, J.D. (2011) 'Association of age and comorbidity with physical function in HIV-infected and uninfected patients: results from the Veterans Aging Cohort Study', *AIDS Patient Care STDS*, 25(1): 13–20.

Power, L., Bell, M. and Freemantle, I. (2010) *A National Study of Ageing and HIV (50 Plus)*, York: Joseph Rowntree Foundation, Available from: http:// www.jrf.org.uk/sites/files/jrf/living-with-HIV-full.pdf

Public Health England (2018) *Progress towards Ending the HIV Epidemic in the United Kingdom: 2018 Report*, London: Public Health England, Available from: https://assets.publishing.service.gov.uk/government/uploads/sys tem/uploads/attachment_data/file/821273/Progress_towards_ending_the _HIV_epidemic_in_the_UK.pdf

Public Health England (2020) *Positive Voices: The National Survey of People Living with HIV: Findings from the 2017 Survey*, London: Public Health England, Available from: https://assets.publishing.service.gov.uk/governm ent/uploads/system/uploads/attachment_data/file/857922/PHE_positive _voices_report_2019.pdf

Rose, N. (2001) 'The politics of life itself', *Theory, Culture & Society*, 18(6): 1–30.

Rosenfeld, D., Anderson, J., Ridge, D., Asboe, D., Catalan, J., Collins, S., Delpech, V., Tuffrey, V. and Porter, T. (2015) *Social Support, Mental Health, and Quality of Life among Older People Living with HIV: Findings from the HIV and Later Life (HALL) Project*, Keele: Keele University.

Smit, M., Brinkman, K., Geerlings, S., Smit, C., Thyagarajan, K., van Sighem, A., de Wolf, F. and Hallett, T.B. (2015) 'Future challenges for clinical care of an ageing population infected with HIV: a modelling study', *The Lancet*, 15(7): 810–18.

Solomon, J. (2007) *Living with 'X': A Body Mapping Journey in the Time of HIV and AIDS. Facilitator's Guide*, Johannesburg: Regional Psychosocial Support Initiative (REPSSI).

Sophia Forum and Terrence Higgins Trust (2018) *Women and HIV: Invisible No Longer. A National Study of Women's Experiences of HIV*, London: Sophia Forum and Terrence Higgins Trust, Available from: http://sophiaforum.net/wp-content/uploads/2018/04/Invisible-No-Longer-full-report-of-a-national-study-of-women-and-HIV.pdf

Stevenson, J. (2022) ' "It feels like my visibility matters": women ageing with HIV overcoming the "violence of invisibility" through community, advocacy and the radical act of care for others', *Women's Health* [online], Available from: https://doi.org/10.1177/17455057221095911

Terrence Higgins Trust (nd) 'Can't Pass It On' [online], Available from: https://www.tht.org.uk/our-work/our-campaigns/cant-pass-it-on

UNAIDS (2018) *Undetectable = Untransmittable: Public Health and HIV Viral Load Suppression*, UNAIDS Explainer [online], Available from: https://www.unaids.org/sites/default/files/media_asset/undetectable-untransmittable_en.pdf

Winston, A. and Underwood, J. (2015) 'Emerging concepts on the use of antiretroviral therapy in older adults living with HIV infection', *Current Opinion in Infectious Diseases*, 28(1): 17–22.

Young, I., Davis, M., Flowers, P. and McDaid, L.M. (2019) 'Navigating HIV citizenship: identities, risks and biological citizenship in the treatment as prevention era', *Health, Risk & Society*, 21(1–2): 1–16.

3

'Everyone is on their own and nobody needs us': women ageing with HIV in Ukraine

Tetyana Semigina, Tetiana Yurochko and Yulia Stopolyanska

Introduction

The population in the world is ageing. People living with HIV are not an exception: globally, from 2000 to 2016, the share of people living with HIV older than 50 increased from 8 to 16 per cent (Autenrieth et al, 2018). This is occurring due to the availability of antiretroviral treatment (ART), because more young people practise safe behaviours and because HIV infection may be acquired later in life (Freeman and Anglewicz, 2012).

In recent years, a substantial body of research has indicated peculiarities of ageing with HIV or being diagnosed HIV at an older age, and the low level of knowledge about HIV among the older population (Orchi et al, 2008; Nardelli et al, 2016; Davis and Elder, 2020). International agencies have suggested programmes to increase the quality of life of mature people living with HIV (UNAIDS, 2013; Global HIV Prevention Coalition, 2020); at the same time, they have highlighted the importance of diagnostic interventions in routine interactions between older people and healthcare providers.

Like many European countries, Ukraine is an ageing society. According to the State Statistics Service of Ukraine, in 2014 the share of the Ukrainian population aged 60 years or over was 21.4 per cent, and forecasts suggest that this will increase to 25 per cent by 2025 and 38 per cent by 2050 (Talko, 2015). Ukraine has a high prevalence of HIV. However, policy programmes, statistics and research are focused primarily on individuals aged 15–49 and children. Information on both HIV prevalence in older adults and their HIV risk behaviours has been lacking. Gender-sensitive HIV services and programmes are rare, and the specific needs of women are not met (Shulga et al, 2015; Demchenko et al, 2017).

This chapter presents findings from a study of the lived experiences of women aged 50 and older living with HIV in three large cities in Ukraine,

Editors' note: This chapter was developed and written before the Russian invasion of Ukraine in 2022.

as well as information obtained from social workers. The UNAIDS (2013) definition of older people living with HIV refers to people 50 years of age or older, and we applied that age threshold in this study. The chapter also highlights the need for Ukrainian government HIV programmes to take account of the needs of older people. The chapter concludes with suggestions for prevention interventions for women ageing with HIV.

Theoretical perspectives

The experiences of HIV-positive older women in Ukraine can be viewed through two conceptual lenses. These are helpful for analysing perceptions of HIV and critically reviewing existing services and programmes, as well as for designing innovative prevention programmes for Ukraine.

First, a structuralist perspective was used to understand the specifics of stigma experienced by women, older people, HIV-positive people or any other group within society. We share Wingood and DiClemente's (2000) view that the structural theory of gender and power (based on existing philosophical concepts of sexual inequality, gender and power imbalance, and considering the gendered relationships between men and women) can be applied to analysis of data. This perspective may help to investigate the multifaceted challenges of HIV-positive older women living in a post-socialist society with many gender stereotypes and restrictions about sexual intimacy (Martsenyuk, 2012; Gradskova and Morell, 2018).

The pro-feminist researchers Bowden and Mummery (2009) and Eyal-Lubling and Krumer-Nevo (2016) point out the possibilities of using a feminist framework to unmask key gender aspects of social stigma and discrimination towards HIV-positive women, to understand 'private as public' and to seek collective measures to solve personal issues. Literature (Bos et al, 2013; Kowalski and Peipert, 2019; Johnson et al, 2021) suggests a clear link between public opinion and stereotypes that lead to self-stigmatisation, internalised stigma or diminishing identities of a woman. From this perspective, a broader process of cultural change in different areas of society is needed to challenge the stigmatisation of HIV-positive older women, and sociopolitical actions are needed on different levels (Dominelli, 2002), as well as gender-specific empowering interventions, especially for women from marginalised groups (Houston, 2016; Gupta, 2000). Such approaches are also reflected in UNAIDS recommendations on gender equality and HIV (UNAIDS, 2010, 2014).

The second lens is related to the concept of healthy ageing (World Health Organization, 2017; Naah et al, 2020). To ensure that ageing is healthy for as many people as possible and to combat marginalisation and discrimination against older persons, the European Union introduced a policy aimed at 'helping people stay in charge of their own lives for as long as possible as they age and, where possible, to contribute to the economy and society' (European Union, 2019, p 9).

Freeman and Anglewicz (2012) provide notable reasons why HIV infection at older ages is an important public health concern: first, adults initiating treatment at the age of 50 or over are significantly more likely to die than those initiating treatment at a younger age; and, second, older infected adults experience higher rates of many non-AIDS-related illnesses than younger infected adults or older uninfected adults. For these reasons, age-specific public health programmes are needed to support healthy ageing, including the prevention of HIV among older persons. These programmes should be system-wide and multisectoral (Valdiserri, 2018; Global HIV Prevention Coalition, 2020) and reflect concerns specific to older persons. Davis and Elder (2020) reveal that older people need more education programmes about HIV, covering topics such as modes of transmission, specifics of disease at different ages, and life changes that can be attributed to disease. This should include education regarding the sexual lives of older persons, which has so far been regarded as a 'blind spot' (Banke-Thomas et al, 2020). Moreover, these actions should be gender specific, as physiological changes in women due to menopause not only cause changes in psycho-emotional and sexual behaviours but also bring a higher risk of infection with sexually transmitted diseases (Thornton et al, 2015).

These two frameworks provide the foundation for our study of older HIV-positive women's personal accounts and can be useful in building a collective, system-wide response to ensure their visibility in HIV prevention programmes.

Background information on HIV in Ukraine

Ukraine has one of the highest HIV prevalence rates in Europe. As of 1 January 2021, the special government registry indicated 144,089 people living with HIV (378.8 per 100,000 population) and 47,788 people with AIDS (125.6 per 100,000 population). During January 2021, 1,001 new cases of HIV, 313 cases of AIDS and 158 AIDS-related deaths were added (Public Health Center, 2021). Registration for HIV-positive people is not compulsory, nor is HIV testing for the wider population. However, testing is highly recommended during pregnancy, so to get relevant medical help, de facto HIV testing is practically obligatory in this context. Dvoriak et al (2019) estimate that only one in six Ukrainians know their HIV status.

The key risk groups defined by the Ukrainian government are: people who inject drugs, sex workers, men who have sex with men, prisoners and sexual partners of key affected populations (Avert, 2019). In 2020, the main mode of HIV transmission was heterosexual intercourse, and women were mostly infected in this way (Public Health Center, 2021). However, up to this point, the HIV-positive population has been dominated by people who inject drugs, as the parenteral route was the most common among those diagnosed with HIV early in the pandemic. Thus, in Ukraine, HIV is mainly portrayed as a 'disease of drug addicts'.

Novak et al (2017) demonstrate that since young people are less likely to be infected, the profile of the overall HIV-positive population is ageing. However, there are no official statistics on the number of people older than 50 living with HIV. Research conducted in 2020 for the Stigma Index, which measures stigma against people with HIV, included 20 per cent of older people (people over 50) in the study sample (Demchenko et al, 2021).

Since mid-2000, people living with HIV have been able to access antiretroviral drugs at special state medical facilities (AIDS centres), whereas social services for this group are still provided by community-based mutual aid organisations, financed mainly through international donor aid.

Methods

The study aimed to develop recommendations for HIV prevention programmes that target post-reproductive women. The methods employed were:

- in-depth interviews with six HIV-positive women (clients in community-based mutual aid organisations for people living with HIV);
- in-depth interviews with six social workers in the field (five were working in the mutual aid organisations and one was from a municipal AIDS centre) – three disclosed, unprompted, that they were HIV-positive;
- a desk review of government programmes to combat and eliminate HIV/AIDS.

The interview guides were developed from an intersectional feminist and social constructionist standpoint. We share Pascal's (2010) idea that through accessing the lived experiences of the participant, a researcher may gain understanding of the meanings and perceptions of the other person's world. The main focus of the approach used in this study was human experience, particularly the implicit and explicit meanings embedded in participants' descriptions of their lives with HIV, including their sexual lives.

The interview guide for clients of mutual aid organisations included questions on the emotional experience of living with HIV, attitudes towards sexual practices and risky sexual behaviours, understanding sexuality and self-identification, the impact of HIV on their social roles, self-stigmatisation and attitudes towards preventive programmes. The interview guide for social workers included the same questions, plus a few questions on their observation of the behaviours of older women living with HIV. All questions were focused around the research objective and were open-ended. The interview approach allowed respondents to direct the conversation and discuss their experiences in their own time and in as much depth as they felt comfortable with.

Nine in-depth interviews were conducted with women aged 50 or older who were living with HIV. All of these women were recruited for interview through community-based mutual aid organisations in three cities in Ukraine (Cherkasy, Dnipro and Kyiv). All were of post-reproductive age – seven were aged between 50 and 52, and two were aged 53 to 56 – and were in menopause. All nine were on ART, though with different levels of adherence. Six women reported that they had experience with injecting drug use. Four disclosed that they had provided commercial sex services, and one of them was still an active sex worker at the time of interview. Eight of the women were working (the retirement age for women in Ukraine is 60 years). Three of these women were social workers (peer-to-peer consultants) in HIV services.

Three additional interviews were carried out with social workers in community-based HIV services. They were all under 50 (30, 38 and 45 years old), and we did not ask about their HIV status. So, overall, we recruited six social workers of different ages, from three cities (three were HIV-positive women in their fifties, and three, whose HIV status was not known, were younger than 50). One of these six worked for a municipal AIDS centre, five were consultants in the community-based mutual aid HIV services. Five of the six social workers had taken part in a previous innovative gender-specific project that one of the researchers (Tetyana Semigina) was involved in and supervised during 2012–15. Information on participants is summarised in Table 3.1.

Interviews were conducted by phone or via online chat, and lasted for around an hour. Relevant ethical procedures were followed. The interviews were transcribed, and thematic analysis (Pascal, 2010) was undertaken by the research team. This chapter includes an overview of the themes that emerged from the study: learning about HIV-positive status; sexual behaviours after learning about HIV-positive status; attitudes of medical personnel and access

Table 3.1: Characteristics of the interviewees (n = 12)

	Clients of HIV community centres	Social workers (peer-to-peer consultants)
HIV-positive	6	At least 3
Aged 50+ (post-reproductive age)	6	3
Experience of drug use	At least 6	At least 6
Experience of providing commercial sex services	At least 4	At least 4
Working at the time of the interview	11	11
Receiving ART	9	9

to consultations on sexual issues; self-evaluation and relations within the immediate environment; and attitudes towards prevention programmes.

The desk review of Ukrainian government regulations to combat and eliminate HIV/AIDS epidemics was intended to critically assess the relevance for older women of current HIV prevention policies. This review covered a number of documents issued in recent years (Cabinet of Ministries of Ukraine, 2019; Ministry of Health of Ukraine, 2019). The objectives were to understand specific interventions and to identify the place of older women in these interventions.

The women's voices

Theme 1: Learning about HIV status

Six out of the nine interviewees who disclosed an HIV-positive status were diagnosed for over 15 years, and the others, less than 3 years. The women learned about their diagnosis in different ways. Most had not experienced symptoms before their diagnosis. Identification of HIV-positive status was mostly accidental, either through routine examination during pregnancy or in response to an offer to be tested by mobile teams. As one respondent recalled:

'It was a total shock for me. I didn't expect that at all. And all my worries were about the future baby. Neither medical doctors nor any other personnel provided me with sufficient consultation or advice. I had just got a paper with red letters – HIV. Later, medical doctors prescribed my antiretroviral treatment; these drugs caused awful side effects. I delivered a baby at the special hospital ward, and due to preventive measures my son is healthy. Later, I learned that my husband was also HIV-positive. I suspect infidelity, that he had been with a prostitute or some other women who were infected.' (Maryna, client, 53)

One respondent stated she had experienced excruciating back pain and a very high fever. It was only when she was diagnosed with opportunistic herpes infection that she asked doctors to refer her for an HIV test as she herself suspected she was HIV-positive.

Providing information on the routes of infection, five women stated that they were infected sexually, three stated that it was due to injecting drug use, and one suspected she had been infected with HIV through a blood transfusion performed in connection with complications during childbirth.

All six social workers said that around 10 per cent of their clients learn of their HIV infection by accident and at an older age.

'People are planning surgery operations or have other hospital treatment, or they have some critical situation when opportunistic co-infection has been added. Older people do not apply for HIV-testing on their own, deliberately.' (Alyona, social worker, 30)

'Family doctors are openly saying that in their view or opinion, it is not necessary to send an adult person to do an HIV test because a particular person lives within family and is socially normal.' (Lyuba, social worker, 50)

'Older women sometimes for two, three or five years are treating different sickness with no definite diagnosis, and medical doctors don't even consider the need for HIV-testing.' (Vira, social worker, 45)

Social workers also pointed out that when interacting with the healthcare system, even in the presence of a clinical picture, diagnosis can take a long time.

Theme 2: Sexual behaviours after learning about HIV-positive status

When discussing their sexual life and behaviours, women first of all mentioned the menopause. Most respondents reported that regular menstruation had been absent for more than a year, but did not mention any symptoms or discomfort. Only one woman noted that for her, the period of age-related hormonal changes had been accompanied by a wide range of symptoms – dizziness, cold and hot flashes, and mood swings being the most concerning. She also noted that "the most discomfort is when these symptoms occur in the most inappropriate moment" (Katya, client, 56).

It is worth quoting another woman who did not belong to a key risk group: "Before the HIV diagnosis, I felt all the symptoms of menopause, menstruation disappeared. At first, I thought for a long time that all the symptoms that preceded HIV – for example, fever, back pain, dizziness, fatigue – were symptoms of menopause. Unfortunately, it wasn't menopause" (Maryna, client, 53). This statement draws attention to the lack of awareness of older women about the symptoms of menopause and those of HIV. It is very important to note that this patient described a fairly trusting and long-lasting relationship with her family doctor.

The women's attitudes to their sexual lives varied substantially. The respondent who was an active commercial sex worker noted: "Two to three partners per day, almost without days off. This is my job, I can't say that the onset of menopause somehow affects my attitude to sexual life" (Olga, client, 51).

During interviews, some women said that finding out about their HIV status limited their sexual intercourse. One explained: "I cannot psychologically overcome the barrier. I have highly developed empathy, so I can't disclose my status, and I can't lie either. Even using a condom is not a sufficient argument for me, even if I know that I do not have a virological load" (Maryna, client, 53).

The women who have experience with drug use stated that they do not feel sexual desire. One described her experience of sexual intercourse as follows: "I don't feel any sexual desire, yet I have to respond to the desire of my partner" (Tamara, client, 54).

Interestingly, none of the participants in the study associated a decrease in sexual desire or sexual discomfort with age-related hormonal changes in the body, and their answers were focused either on HIV status as a barrier to a full sexual life or on the experience of risky behaviours.

None of the participants who said they had sex reported using condoms. One of the women with experience of drug use shared in her story:

'When I found out about my status, I immediately informed my [now] ex-husband. He did the test and was healthy. I suggested that he use condoms, but he didn't pay attention and we didn't use protection during sex. I kicked out my husband four years ago, I don't know what's wrong with him now.' (Tamara, client, 54)

Moreover, they expressed unwillingness to disclose their HIV status to casual partners. A commercial sex worker related: "I use condoms if the client wants, and I don't mention HIV" (Olga, client, 51).

Women avoid discussing issues of sexuality, considering this topic 'girlish', not proper for their age and thus their social status. Another participant (Maryna, client 53) noted that sexuality "is when a woman can solve all issues through sexual relations". Yet another (Katya, client 56) considered sexuality to be related to the hormonal system and health in general; if these are good, then a person possesses sexuality. The women with drug experience felt quite uncomfortable during this part of interview and spoke mostly about sexual intercourse.

All women were asked whether they had heard of pre-exposure or post-exposure prophylaxis, but only one woman, who had experience of commercial sex work and is now a social worker at a mutual aid organisation, responded that she had. She mentioned, however, that "so far in my life, it has not been useful to me" (Lyuba, social worker, 50).

Summing up this theme, it is worth stressing that despite the fact that the main route of infection is heterosexual contact, some participants had unprotected sex and some were unlikely to report their HIV status to irregular partners. At the same time, some women deliberately limited sexual intercourse due to a conscious reluctance or fear of infecting a partner, while others did not feel sexual desire.

Theme 3: Attitudes of medical personnel and access to consultations about sexual issues

The HIV-positive women trusted their main providers – including medical doctors specialising in AIDS and family doctors – for issues related to the provision of medical care. Among the factors contributing to open communication, all interviewees agreed that the most important is acceptance and understanding. The willingness of doctors to always be available and ready to help was also mentioned as one of the key elements of a trusting relationship.

All study participants living with HIV used ART. All six social workers observed that older HIV-positive women demonstrate the same level of treatment adherence as younger HIV-positive women. They also observed that HIV-positive women who do not belong to key risk groups are more responsible about taking drugs as prescribed, and they go for examinations on a regular basis; they also monitor their health outside of issues related to HIV. Women from key risk groups reported that their adherence to ART was irregular, and they gave reasons relating to individual choice. One explained, "I may be asleep, or I may feel like missing a pill" (Olga, client, 51), and another said, "I may be taking it regularly, but I had treatment interruptions due to side effects caused by ART" (Tamara, client, 54). It is worth emphasising that none of the women reported barriers to accessing ART or lack availability of drugs.

Interviews revealed institutional stigma towards women because of their HIV status and because of their age, with staff in different medical facilities demonstrating negative attitudes and behaviours.

'Medical doctors are asking more fees for their services than from other patients – because of risks.' (Katya, client, 56)

'I was not aware that I have a right not to disclose my status. Medical doctors threatened me with a criminal case.' (Tamara, client, 54)

'Doctors and nurses discuss the HIV status of their patients with everyone in the city.' (Lyuba, social worker, 50)

The women were wary of discussing their sexual lives with doctors. All respondents expressed the view that they would discuss this topic only when necessary. Reasons for this selective communication are given in the following comments:

'Stigma is very pressing. Medicine is moving forward, but doctors are not.' (Anna, social worker, 38)

'Discrimination and stigma are there and it is very noticeable. Some doctors look at me like a leper, but I don't care. I talk about my status to all doctors, because it is important to get treated. Not everyone wants to help, so I do not apply without a recommendation.' (Katya, client, 56)

'I never talked about it with my infectious disease specialist. Apparently he thinks I'm not interested. And he is a young guy. Well, maybe, I would talk, but dryly and formally.' (Olga, client, 51)

In sum, while women ageing with HIV have trusting relationships with main healthcare providers, they do not trust all medical staff and avoid discussing issues related to their sexual lives.

Theme 4: Self-evaluation and relations within the immediate environment

The social workers who were interviewed stressed that women who belong to key risk groups seldom self-refer to mutual aid HIV services, because they feel ashamed and want to avoid being associated with the HIV community. One commented: "Women have the feeling of shame, especially in front of family or friends. This is due to the misunderstanding that this [contacting HIV] may happen to anyone" (Anna, social worker, 38).

The stories of HIV-positive women demonstrate low self-esteem and self-stigmatisation.

'I am a beautiful woman, I have all the makings, but I do not feel that inner confidence and my self-esteem is gone.' (Maryna, client, 53)

'I can't afford to find a normal job, because I can't feel stress and tension. I want to find an opportunity to work at home and be creative. I am not sure I can find such a job with my age and my status.' (Tamara, client, 54)

'What is the sense of living being an older person, a woman and HIV-positive. Three negative, toxic features that are spoiling my life. Of course, it's my personal fault that I am who I am today.' (Katya, client, 56)

Self-stigmatisation was also evident when women discussed the concept of female sexuality. Most respondents did not identify with the concept, and some even aggressively denied it.

Interviewees also revealed that feelings of self-stigma were exacerbated by the stigma and discrimination that they experience from their immediate environment and society.

'Nerves and worries make life very difficult. Very bad relationship with my family, they did not accept my status. I have to rely only on myself.' (Katya, client, 56)

'My son and his family do not accept me. We have a very tense relationship, although we live in the same apartment.' (Maryna, client, 53)

'I have feelings of depression and lack of hope for understanding. Fear that they will leave you. Everyone is on their own and nobody needs us.' (Tanya, client, 52)

Even the social workers, regardless of their own HIV status, revealed impacts on their close environment due to their professional association with people who are HIV-positive. For example, neighbours stopped communicating with them when they learned about their work in HIV services.

For some of the HIV-positive women interviewed, their HIV status did not create barriers for communicating with their partners. However, a few experienced gender-based violence after their diagnosis. Among the specific manifestations of this violence, clients and social workers mentioned disclosure of status and physical and sexual assault. One said: "Partners are disclosing the status of women. Previously I thought that a man had such a right. I felt myself rather dirty because of HIV" (Lyuba, social worker, 50).

In this study, all HIV-positive respondents focused on their, or other women's, feelings of shame, self-blame and anxiety associated with the discovery of HIV-positive status. There were many stories of family and relatives failing to accept the women because of their status, and some of the women even considered themselves "dirty", "worthless". There was also concern about the effect of stigma and discrimination on patients' accessing care.

Theme 5: Attitudes towards prevention programmes

Participants in the study identified possible preventive measures, such as the expansion of information programmes for the public and training and internships for primary care physicians. Mandatory testing was another option put forward.

'People need information. They need to know and understand what it is. HIV is a closed topic. We need to educate society.' (Lyuba, social worker, 50)

'We need a social programme. People need to talk about it. They need more knowledge, mutual help and support groups, trainings.' (Tamara, client, 54)

'People need to understand that life does not end because of status. It just changes, goes differently.' (Katya, client, 56)

'Family doctors need to undergo training in AIDS centres. They need to see that we are ordinary people.' (Olga, client, 51)

'Mandatory testing should be enshrined in the law. It has to be talked about openly.' (Alyona, social worker, 30)

In terms of reaching older women for preventive work, social workers mentioned that the best channels for communication are family doctors and special public announcements on television and online. Moreover, according to social workers, older women do not engage with prevention programmes that target younger people, as they do not view their HIV as a 'disease of youth' or 'disease of risky youth'.

'Invisibility' of older people in government programmes

Currently, HIV/AIDS is identified as a priority issue for public health and social care policy in Ukraine. HIV/AIDS policy covers a broad range of interventions across prevention, treatment, and care and support for people living with HIV/AIDS.

In assessing the national healthcare system with regard to readiness to implement interventions aimed at containing the spread of HIV, it is worth noting the legal framework that has developed. With the support of international and national stakeholders, legal documents have been approved and form the basis for the implementation of testing, treatment and prevention strategies (including provision of medication) as well as social support services for people at high risk of HIV. At the same time, the current national intervention programmes (Parliament of Ukraine, 2019; Ministry of Health of Ukraine, 2019) are underdeveloped with regard to older people living with HIV. For instance, the practice of routine HIV testing among older people is not singled out as an intervention for control of the HIV epidemic.

Older people are included in state interventions mostly as part of the general population; thus, they are viewed only in the context of other groups, not considered as a separate group with particular needs. The formation of public policy in different areas does not take into account the specific characteristics and needs of different groups in the context of physical and mental conditions. To improve the effectiveness of government programmes, it will be important to rethink the categorisation of key risk groups and to identify older people as a separate group, based on their particular experiences.

It is also important to emphasise that the needs of post-reproductive women living with HIV have not been addressed in government measures to contain the epidemic. Lack of awareness is evident at the primary points of interaction of the healthcare system (infectious disease doctors and family doctors) with this group of people. Services for older women with HIV are not aimed at improving their quality of life, whether in terms of control over their physiological state outside of their HIV status or in terms of providing psycho-emotional support. Our analysis of the current national legal framework confirms that approaches to epidemic control need to be adjusted in order to integrate the needs of older people into national policy. As already mentioned, older people, especially women, are seen in the context of either the general population or key risk groups. Current policies do not take account of the needs of this group or the profile of risk groups among older persons.

Concluding remarks and recommendations

This conclusion highlights some key points raised by the findings and then draws out recommendations for prevention interventions targeting older women living with HIV.

First of all, the findings reflect a complicated picture in terms of gender roles. In Ukraine, an older woman is expected to play the social role of grandmother (*babysia* in Ukrainian) who cares for her family and primarily her grandchildren. *Babysia* should be a model of 'good behaviour' and a 'perfect housekeeper' as well as holding religious beliefs. At the same time, the social value of older women is rather low, as is their self-esteem (Kuhta, 2019). Older women are perceived as powerless and asexual creatures, and talking about their sexuality is 'inappropriate'. Our study contradicts these gendered perceptions of the social norms of ageing.

Second, while research for the Stigma Index (Demchenko et al, 2021) indicates a gradual decrease in the level of stigma and discrimination against people living with HIV in Ukraine, in our study, HIV-positive respondents revealed feelings of shame and anxiety associated with the discovery of their status. Some women considered themselves 'dirty' and 'punished'.

Third, trust is key to women's relationship with healthcare providers and their willingness to talk about sexual health. More than half of the participants had an active sex life. However, as they tended to have only one contact within the healthcare system that they trusted, the women did not see it as acceptable to discuss sexual issues with them and did not feel comfortable doing so. Similar results were reported in a survey of clients at a community social service for older persons (Karkach and Semigina, 2021). At the same time, some women said they would be open to talking about sex if a specialist initiated a conversation. From the perspective of services, doctors' awareness of the need to discuss these issues with older women is insufficient.

Fourth, the findings suggest low awareness among older women about HIV and risk. The study reveals that older people do not consider themselves to be at risk for sexually transmitted diseases and do not rate the risk of HIV transmission as high if they engage in risky sexual practices. This is confirmed by the low level of commitment to using protection.

Fifth, the desk review and interviews confirm that in Ukraine the needs of older women living with HIV are unmet and not integrated properly in government or community programmes to combat HIV, as recommended by international organisations.

The limitations of this small-scale qualitative study are evident, particularly as the social situation in Ukraine is rather dynamic and evolving. The qualitative design inevitably leads to certain selectivity, and the opinions of participants might differ from the wider population of older women living with HIV. Moreover, the HIV-positive women in the study were in the lower age range of this population.

In some cases, respondents provided ambivalent statements in their narratives. However, such spaces of ambivalence are common for the representatives of marginalised groups and could be linked to the uncertainties and disputes in biomedicine and society that are discussed by Patton (2007).

Another sensitive issue is the researchers' empathy towards the women. The close 'distance' between study participants and researchers could be regarded as 'normal' in social work, as well as standing for social justice (Dominelli, 2002). However, the closeness of relationships also introduces concern about interpretation of findings.

The findings from the study allow us to recommend the inclusion of adults aged 50 and over in HIV/AIDS research and prevention efforts. There should be a specific focus on women of post-reproductive age. Prevention programmes can draw from experiences in other countries (UNAIDS, 2013; Valdiserri, 2018; Banke-Thomas et al, 2020; Davis and Elder, 2020) and should focus on healthy and active ageing (European Union, 2019). Options include:

- a nationwide public information campaign aimed at raising awareness of contracting HIV in older age and ageing with HIV, with topics such as safe sexual intercourse for older persons (using 'ordinary' women and family doctors as key channels for sharing messages);
- macro-level education work among the target group of older people, aiming to reduce risky behaviours, to highlight the need for HIV testing and to downgrade the stigma associated with HIV-positive status;

- piloting and national dissemination of in-depth training for social workers on the physiological, psychological and social aspects of HIV for older women;
- training for family doctors on the nature of HIV in older age and the need for HIV testing for older people, and training for medical doctors in AIDS centres on how to provide consultations for older HIV-positive women about their sexual lives;
- actions in the local communities worst affected by HIV, to provide age-friendly services for people ageing with HIV and other older people.

Innovative empowering programmes for women ageing with HIV are needed to overcome self-stigmatisation. Innovations must focus on improving women's self-esteem and livelihoods. Such pro-feminist programmes have worked well in Ukraine for middle-aged women with small children (Semigina and Tymoshenko, 2016) and, with certain amendments, could be used to address service gaps in the support of older women living with HIV.

Through an age-friendly innovative intervention, case managers could work directly with mature women living with HIV to develop individualised plans that outline actions to address personal challenges. These actions might include referrals to psychosocial support services, arranging medical consultations or providing assistance to access social welfare. Women could also participate in group interventions to receive mutual support and gain skills to address common challenges, such as self-confidence, stress management, relations with relatives and partners, conflict resolution, personal health and women's rights.

Global and European policy actors as well as professional associations could provide specific guidelines on how to work with older people living with HIV. Such guidelines might include how to introduce information campaigns for the broader community of older people in order to prevent HIV transmission, change perceptions of HIV as a disease of young people and transform discriminatory public perceptions of people living with HIV. National policymakers and local communities might use these transnational recommendations to improve targeted services and develop culturally appropriate initiatives. Also, best practice for effective age- and gender-specific multidisciplinary medical and psychosocial interventions for older people living with HIV could be developed, tested and shared. Evidence and verified information from different countries could be provided via UNAIDS or the World Health Organization.

Of course, building up effective global, national and local preventive programmes to minimise new infection among adults in mid and later life requires detailed information about age patterns of HIV prevalence and risky sexual behaviours, the most likely mode of HIV transmission.

References

Autenrieth, C.S., Beck, E.J., Stelzle, D., Mallouris, C., Mahy, M. and Ghys, P. (2018) 'Global and regional trends of people living with HIV aged 50 and over: estimates and projections for 2000–2020', *PLoS ONE* [online], 13(11): e0207005. doi: 10.1371/journal.pone.0207005

Avert (2019) 'HIV and AIDS in Ukraine' [online], Available from: https://www.avert.org/professionals/hiv-around-world/eastern-europe-central-asia/ukraine

Banke-Thomas, A., Olorunsaiye, C.Z. and Yaya, S. (2020) '"Leaving no one behind" also includes taking the elderly along concerning their sexual and reproductive health and rights: a new focus for *Reproductive Health*', *Reproductive Health* [online], 17(1): 101. doi: 10.1186/s12978-020-00944-5

Bos, A.E.R., Pryor, J.B., Reeder, G. and Stutterheim, S.E. (2013) 'Stigma: advances in theory and research', *Basic and Applied Social Psychology*, 35(1): 1–9.

Bowden, P. and Mummery, J. (2009) *Understanding Feminism*, London: Routledge.

Cabinet of Ministries of Ukraine (2019) On approval of State strategy of combating HIV-infection/AIDS, tuberculosis and viral hepatitis for the period till 2030. [online], Available from: https://zakon.rada.gov.ua/laws/show/1415-2019- [Accessed 5 May 2021].

Davis, T.E.K. and Elder, M.A. (2020) 'HIV knowledge and references for HIV prevention among older adults living in the community', *Gerontology and Geriatric Medicine* [online], 6. https://journals.sagepub.com/doi/10.1177/2333721420927948

Demchenko, I., Varban, M., Bulyga, N. and Holtsas, L. (2017) 'Gender-sensitive harm reduction interventions in Ukraine: clients' perspective', *Visnyk Akademiyi pratsi, sotsial'nykh vidnosyn i turyzmu*, 3: 12–25.

Demchenko, I., Skokova, L. and Bulyga, N. (2021) 'Index of Stigma toward People Living with HIV 2.0', *100% Life* [online], Available from: https://network.org.ua/wp-content/uploads/2021/02/INDEKS-STYGMY-LYU DEJ-YAKI-ZHYVUT-Z-VIL-2.0-1-1.pdf

Dominelli, L. (2002) *Feminist Social Work Theory and Practice*, London: Palgrave.

Dvoriak, S., Karagodina, O., Chtenguelov, V. and Pykalo, I. (2019) 'Ten years of opioid agonist therapy implementation experience in Ukraine. What further? (second part)', *Visnyk Akademiyi pratsi, sotsial'nykh vidnosyn i turyzmu*, 1: 30–41.

European Union (2019) *Ageing Europe: Looking at the Lives of Older People in the EU*, Luxembourg: Publications Office of the European Union.

Eyal-Lubling, R. and Krumer-Nevo, M. (2016) 'Feminist social work: practice and theory of practice', *Social Work*, 61(3): 245–54.

Freeman, E. and Anglewicz, P. (2012) 'HIV prevalence and sexual behaviour at older ages in rural Malawi', *International Journal of STD & AIDS*, 23(7): 490–6.

Global HIV Prevention Coalition (2020) *Implementation of the HIV Prevention 2020 Road Map: Fourth Progress Report*, Geneva: UNAIDS, Available from: https://www.unaids.org/sites/default/files/media_asset/fourth-ann ual-progress-report-global-hiv-prevention-coalition_en.pdf

Gradskova, Y. and Morell, I. (2018) *Gendering Postsocialism: Old Legacies, New Hierarchies*, London: Routledge.

Gupta, G.R. (2000) 'Gender, sexuality, and HIV/AIDS: the what, the why, and the how', *Canadian HIV/AIDS Policy and Law Review*, 5(4): 86–93.

Houston, S. (2016) 'Empowering the "shamed" self: recognition and critical social work', *Journal of Social Work*, 16(1): 3–21.

Johnson, S., Brough, M. and Darracott, R. (2021) 'Unmasking depression: challenging structural oppression whilst recognising individual agency', *Qualitative Social Work*, 20(3): 738–54.

Karkach, A.V. and Semigina, T.V. (2021) 'Adult love: sexual activity in elderly', in *The Driving Force of Science and Trends in Its Development: II International Scientific and Theoretical Conference, Volume 1*, pp 42–4.

Kowalski, R.M. and Peipert, A. (2019) 'Public- and self-stigma attached to physical versus psychological disabilities', *Stigma and Health*, 4(20): 136–42.

Kuhta, M.P. (2019) *Social Potential of Older People in Modern Ukrainian Society*, PhD dissertation, Institute of Sociology, Kyiv.

Martsenyuk, T. (2012) 'The state of the LGBT community and homophobia in Ukraine', *Problems of Post-Communism*, 59(2): 51–62.

Ministry of Health of Ukraine (2019) 'On approval of order on the provision of services for the representatives of the more risky groups for contracting HIV' [online], Available from: https://zakon.rada.gov.ua/laws/show/ z0855-19#Text

Naah, F.L., Njong, A.M. and Kimengsi, J.N. (2020) 'Determinants of active and healthy ageing in Sub-Saharan Africa: evidence from Cameroon', *International Journal of Environmental Research and Public Health* [online], 17(9): 3038. doi:10.3390/ijerph17093038

Nardelli, G.G., Malaquias, B.S.S., Gaudenci, E.M., Ledic, C.S., Azevedo, N.F., Martins, V.E. and Santos, A.S. (2016) 'Knowledge about the human immunodeficiency syndrome among elders in a unit for the care of the elderly', *Revista Gaúcha de Enfermagem* [online], 37(spe): e2016-0039, Available from: https://doi.org/10.1590/1983-1447.2016.esp.2016-0039

Novak, Y., Sorokalit, A., Kutinska, O. and Neduzhko, O. (2017) *Regional Project on Triangulation of Data Related to Combating HIV Infection in Lviv Region*, Kyiv, Ukraine: Alliance for Public Health.

Orchi, N., Balzano, R. and Scognamiglio, P. (2008) 'Ageing with HIV: newly diagnosed older adults in Italy', *AIDS Care*, 20(4): 419–25.

Pascal, J. (2010) 'Phenomenology as a research method for social work contexts: understanding the lived experience of cancer survival', *Currents: New Scholarship in the Human Services*, 9(2): 1–23.

Patton, C. (2007) 'Bullets, balance, or both: medicalisation in HIV treatment', *The Lancet*, 369(9562): 706–7.

Public Health Center (2021) 'Statistics on officially registered cases of HIV infection, AIDS and death cases associated with AIDS in January, 2021', Available from: www.phc.org.ua

Semigina, T. and Tymoshenko, N. (2016) '"I feel alive!": developing an empowering intervention for HIV-positive women in Ukraine', *Social Dialogue*, 14: 28–31.

Shulga, L., Varban, M., Yaremenko, Y. and Demchenko, I. (2015) *Summary of Results of Formative Study of Gender-Oriented Projects and Services in the Harm Reduction*, Kyiv: Alliance for Public Health, Available from: http://aph.org.ua/wp-content/uploads/2016/08/Resume-eng.pdf

Talko, M. (2015) 'Social background of pension reform in Ukraine', *Economic Analysis*, 19(1): 212–17.

Thornton, K., Jervenak, J. and Neal-Perry, G. (2015) 'Menopause and sexuality', *Endocrinology and Metabolism Clinics of North America*, 44(3): 649–61.

UNAIDS (2010) *Agenda for Accelerated Country Action for Women, Girls, Gender Equality and HIV: Operational Plan for the UNAIDS Action Framework*, Geneva: UNAIDS.

UNAIDS (2013) *HIV and Ageing: A Special Supplement to the UNAIDS Report on the Global AIDS Epidemic 2013*, Geneva: UNAIDS, Available from: https://www.unaids.org/sites/default/files/media_asset/20131101_JC2563_hiv-and-aging_en_0.pdf

UNAIDS (2014) *Gender Assessment Tool: Towards a Gender-Transformative HIV Response*, Geneva: UNAIDS.

Valdiserri, R.O. (2018) 'The evolution of HIV prevention programming: moving from intervention to system', *AIDS Education and Prevention*, 30(3): 187–98.

Wingood, G.M. and DiClemente, R.J. (2000) 'Application of the theory of gender and power to examine HIV-related exposures, risk factors, and effective interventions for women', *Health Education & Behavior*, 27(5): 539–65.

World Health Organization (2017) *Global Strategy and Action Plan on Ageing and Health*, Geneva: World Health Organization.

PART II

Gay and bisexual men

4

Chemsex among gay men living with HIV aged over 45 in England and Italy: sociality and pleasure in times of undetectability

Cesare Di Feliciantonio

Introduction

> 'Sometimes I end up doing it [sex under the influence of drugs] on a midweek afternoon with maybe just one bloke from Grindr, sometimes it's ten people on a weekend ... there are drugs and Viagra, you know it's gonna be fun.' (Ben, 55–65, Manchester)

The use of recreational drugs to enhance and facilitate sex, mostly among men who have sex with men is now commonly referred as 'chemsex'. Despite originating in the London scene in relation to the use of GHB/GHL, often referred to as 'G', crystal methamphetamine, often referred to as 'tina' or 'T', and mephedrone, often referred to as 'mcat' in England (Stuart, 2013), the term 'chemsex' has now travelled well beyond the English context and is used also in contexts where other recreational drugs might be used for sex. According to social theorist Kane Race (2015, 2018), chemsex is defined not just by the use of recreational drugs (combined with sexuopharmaceuticals such as Viagra and Cialis in their patented or generic versions) during the sexual encounter, but also by what he calls the 'infrastructures of the sexual encounter' (2015, p 254), including 3G (the standard at the time), Wi-Fi and hook-up apps (for example, Grindr). The quotation at the beginning of this chapter, from the interview with Ben, highlights the significance of these elements in shaping the experience of chemsex.

The use of drugs for sexual pleasure within gay communities is not new. As recently argued by Florêncio (2021, p 8), 'drugs, in some form or another, have been a part of queer culture for a very long time, and are certainly present in a lot of the 20th- and 21st-century queer cultural outputs'. For him, it is important to acknowledge the histories of sexualised drug use 'as part of the history of a subculture' (2021, p 10) that includes rituals of drug consumption than can be traced back to the early years of the AIDS epidemic. These histories are often removed from official documents (for example, laws, regulations) and mainstream narratives around drugs that build 'drugs' as the symbol of the moral decay of society and reduce any form of drug consumption to (individual) 'weakness' and/or 'addiction' (Dennis, 2019). Recent mediatic discourse on chemsex tends to rely on the same script, mixed to old homophobic ideas, framing specific gay subjects as dangerous, irresponsible and bringing death (Lovelock, 2018). From a public health perspective, chemsex has been mostly framed as a pathological issue derived from internalised homophobia, drug addiction and HIV-related stigma, and requiring professional intervention because it is associated with higher rates of sexually transmitted infections (for example, Kirby and Thornbur-Dunwell, 2013; Stuart, 2013; Bourne et al, 2015; Bryant et al, 2018). Rejecting pathologising and individualising analyses of this practice, scholars in social and cultural studies have oriented 'critical chemsex studies' (Møller and Hakim, 2021) along three main lines of enquiry: going beyond the risk paradigm (for example, Drysdale et al, 2020); the sociocultural and political economy dimension of chemsex (for example, Hakim, 2019); and the focus on play and pleasure to understand gay intimacy and sociality (for example, Pienaar et al, 2020).

Situated at the intersection between the second and the third lines of enquiry conceptualised by Møller and Hakim (2021), this chapter focuses on an underexplored dimension within the social science literature on chemsex: ageing with HIV. Even though public health literature, service providers and practitioners usually refer to those aged over 50 when discussing 'ageing with HIV', this chapter slightly expands that definition in an analysis of the relationship between the life course and engagement with chemsex in the narratives of self-identified gay men living with HIV aged over 45 – a group usually referred to as 'midlife' (Simpson, 2013) – who practise chemsex in England and Italy. From a generational perspective, the chapter concerns the narratives of the so called 'AIDS-2 Generation' (Hammack et al, 2018), also defined as 'insulated from the epidemic' (Tester, 2018) – that is, the generation that contracted HIV after the peak of the epidemic in the Global North in the 1980s and therefore had access to effective antiretroviral therapy (ART). The sexual lives of people living with HIV have been mostly studied in terms of prevention, 'risk-taking' and health promotion, overlooking the dimension of pleasure (a central component for one's well-being). Against this trend, the chapter highlights the role of chemsex as a source of pleasure for research participants, therefore contributing to a better understanding of how drugs can help people 'to experiment with what the body can do' (Piennar et al, 2020, p 4). This is a fundamental task for scholars and practitioners willing to promote (even within a harm-reduction perspective) the well-being of people living with HIV, a social group with a long history of stigma that has made the HIV-positive body somehow 'untouchable' (Chapman, 2000), leading to a negative self-perception of one's own body.

The results of the analysis presented in the chapter show how participants frame their engagement with chemsex as driven by the quest for sociality combined with a rediscovery of sexual pleasure and an improved sense of comfort with their bodies resulting from the emergence of the paradigm of undetectability – that is, the now established medical knowledge that people living with HIV with an undetectable viral load who adhere to ART regularly cannot transmit the virus (for a review on the implications of undetectability over gay and bisexual men's lives, see Brown and Di Feliciantonio, 2022). However, the chapter argues that in order to fully understand the relationship between chemsex and the life course for this generation of gay men living with HIV, it is necessary to consider two more processes that are central to their experiences: intergenerationality and intersectionality. The adoption of an intergenerational and intersectional perspective complicates participants' narratives, highlighting tensions and ambivalences within their engagement with chemsex. Against romantic narratives of chemsex, the chapter shows how this practice can generate *both* positive feelings around pleasure and sociality *and* uncomfortable situations; moreover, it shows how chemsex can favour *both* the (sexual) encounter with social difference (for example, intergenerational) *and* the reproduction of social inequalities around, among others, age, class, race, performance of masculinity and body size.

The remainder of the chapter is organised as follows. In the next section, I present the theoretical framework, connecting social and cultural studies analyses of chemsex with the concepts of life course, intergenerationality and intersectionality, which have shaped data analysis. The research methods are then described. Next, I analyse participants' self-narratives of chemsex, highlighting the importance of undetectability for understanding their renewed comfort with their bodies and sex itself while also showing the central role of intergenerational relations behind their engagement with chemsex. Then an intersectional perspective is adopted to analyse the role of several markers of social identity (notably class and economic resources; homeownership or, more generally, independent living; race; the performance of masculinity; and body size) in shaping the experience of chemsex for the research participants. Finally, in the conclusion, I discuss the limitations of the study in relation to the age of participants, emphasising the need for future research to look at the relationship between sex, drugs and the experience of ageing with HIV among those who are aged over 65.

Chemsex and ageing with HIV: life course, intergenerationality and intersectionality

Against the medical framing of chemsex as an individual journey through trauma and destructive behaviours (for example, Brennan et al, 2007), critical scholars across the social sciences and cultural studies have produced a more complex, relational and social understanding of this practice. For Race, chemsex can be theorised as 'culture', that is, 'a cluster of activities and practices that are meaningful for participants with their own organising logics and relative coherence; a significant source of pleasure, connection, eroticism and intimacy – notwithstanding the known dangers' (2015, p 256). For Race, the sexual spaces produced by chemsex often lead to community formation. In his view, chemsex results from considering sex as play within online gay communities, opening new possibilities for pleasure and experimentation. In a more recent co-authored paper (Pienaar et al, 2020), Race and colleagues, aiming to challenge the view of drugs as inherently harmful and risky without considering the other phenomena composing individual and collective lives, explore how the use of drugs allow research participants to alter their bodily experience (in the case of people who might struggle with their own bodies, such as trans people) and experiment with new and unimagined erotic practices. Building on Race's work, Hakim (2019) analyses the rise of chemsex in London as part of a series of conjunctural dynamics, including the diffusion of digital technologies. Opposing the panic behind chemsex in public discourse in Britain, he defines chemsex in London as 'a way for some, largely migrant, gay and bisexual men to experience a sense of collectivity' (Hakim, 2019, p 253). Taken together, these contributions offer the possibility to understand the generative character of chemsex beyond pathologising and individualising tendencies. Although increasing efforts are being devoted to expanding the analytical breath of chemsex research in order to include more subjects and 'scenes' in a dynamic perspective (Pienaar et al, 2020; Drysdale, 2021), some markers of social difference remain underexplored in chemsex social science research, age being one of them.

In order to contribute to a better understanding of the ways age(ing) shapes engagement with chemsex among men living with HIV, it is important to consider the three main processes that, according to social science scholars, shape the experience of age(ing): life course, intergenerationality and intersectionality (for example, Hopkins and Pain, 2007; Ferrer et al, 2017; Brotman et al, 2020).

The life course perspective places individuals in time-space contexts on the assumption that every individual develops their own life trajectory, with personal trajectories affecting each other (Elder, 1994). According to this framework, each individual trajectory is situated in a broader historical and geographical context, and therefore the life course results from the interplay between agency and structure: individual decisions are influenced by circumstances and by the encounter with other lives. The life course perspective has been used across the social sciences in multiple ways, from studying life transitions (for example, childhood, motherhood) to examining the role of historical events over life trajectories (Mayer, 2009). Thinking about life transitions is particularly important when analysing LGBTIQ lives because it allows us to go beyond normative ideas of life stages based on heteronormative temporalities (for example, Halberstam, 2005). Moreover, its use highlights the inadequacy of chronological age indicators to identify people as 'young' or 'old' (Settersten and Mayer, 1997). The life course approach has also been used in HIV social science research, mainly in relation to risk (for example, Mojola et al, 2015; Ruark et al, 2016). According to Rosenfeld et al (2012), a life course approach is the most suitable for understanding the life experiences of the gay cohort in the baby boomer generation, because they went through the gay rights movement first and the HIV/AIDS epidemic peak later. In their words, 'regardless of their own HIV status, gay male baby boomers are aging in a context strongly shaped by these heavy losses and within heavily depleted social networks, with as yet unknown consequences for later life' (Rosenfeld et al, 2012, p 257).

Intergenerationality has emerged as a response to the compartmentalisation of research on age, shifting the focus from either young people or older people to interactions and relations between/among families, generations and networks, and emphasising how society is ordered according to 'age-appropriate' expectations and behaviours (Hagestad and Uhlenberg, 2005; Vanderbeck, 2007). The intergenerational perspective acknowledges how the experience of age is not simply affected by other age groups, but defined and produced through the interaction with other groups. The importance of intergenerational relations to understanding access to gay venues and feelings about a presumed 'gay community' has been explored by a vast amount of social science scholarship (for example, Heaphy, 2007, 2009; Slevin and Linneman, 2010; Simpson, 2013, 2014). For instance, Simpson's analysis of Manchester's gay village reveals that 'the bar "scene" represents a sensorium of pleasures where the "gay gaze" can operate in more benign or affirmative ways not always linked to ageist scrutiny or sexual desire and can include cross-generational intimacies' (2013, p 284). Intergenerationality plays an important role in the experience of living with HIV beyond the discussion on a presumed 'post-AIDS' generation (Walker, 2020); for instance, because the virus is associated with 'risky' practices, it is usually supposed to be contracted at a young age, leaving those who contract it later in life confused and lacking support (Heidari, 2016).

Academically, the concept of intersectionality was introduced by Crenshaw (1991) in her work on Black women's employment experiences; however, she pointed to the potential of intersectionality in 'mediating the tensions between assertions of multiple identity and the ongoing necessity of group politics' (p 1296). Since then, intersectionality has become a hegemonic concept across the social sciences (Davis, 2008). In response to the common focus on the 'triad' of class/gender/race as the most important factors defining one's experience, critical scholarship has stressed the need to question a broader range of identity markers, including health status and its impact (Nash, 2008; Dhamoon, 2011; Brown, 2012). In a recent review paper on intersectionality in social geography, Hopkins (2019) warns against the Whitening of the use of this concept (for example, considering gender but not race). Following Collins and Bilge (2016), his review (Hopkins, 2019, p 942) highlights three core points behind intersectionality: social context (for example, historical contexts and institutions); relationality (that is, identities are not fixed and stable, but built relationally); and a focus on complexity, inequalities, power and social justice. The chapter builds on Hopkins' critique by combining the analysis of social context (chemsex as a subcultural practice), relationality (the importance of the intergenerational encounter) and power dynamics (how the practice of chemsex can reproduce specific inequalities and power relations while also favouring encounter and pleasure).

Methods

Methodologically, the chapter draws on research conducted as part of a comparative transnational project (2018–20) on the lives of different generations of gay men living with HIV in England and Italy. The project relied on different methods (a survey; biographic interviews; interviews with service providers; media discourse analysis), but the present chapter is based only on the biographic interviews with gay men living with HIV. A total of 59 biographic interviews were completed across the two countries; the analysis included in this chapter focuses on participants who made reference to practising chemsex (25 out of 59 participants). Given the focus of this chapter on ageing with HIV, most of the data informing the analysis result from interviews with nine research participants who practise chemsex and are aged over 45 (six belong to the 45–54 age group and three to the 55–64 age group). Interviews were conducted in person by the author in two Italian cities (Bologna and Milan) and three English ones (Leicester, London and Manchester). Participants were recruited through ads in online hook-up apps and websites (Bareback Real Time, Grindr), via attendance at dozens of meetings and events designed for gay men living with HIV, and by snowball sampling. The study received ethical approval from both the host university (University of Leicester) and the funder (European Commission) through two separate review processes. All participants provided informed written consent. Whenever possible, interviews were based on the guidelines of the biographic narrative interpretive method (see Wengraf, 2001); that is, the interview was realised in two parts. In the first part, the participant was only asked a very broad question about his life, so he was actually free to talk about whatever he wanted, for as long as he wanted; there was no moderation from my part. The second interview followed the more traditional model of the semi-structured interview, with the questions based on what was (or was not) said in the first interview. As expected, the interviews diverged greatly in length (from 62 to 341 minutes) and topics covered. Participants were free to use objects or pictures that they felt the need for. In line with ethical guidelines, the interviews were fully anonymous (that is, any personal information making them identifiable was removed; other characteristics, such as age and occupation, were classified under general categories), and the participants were given the opportunity to choose a pseudonym or code. Interview transcripts were coded in a three stage-process. The first stage was based on a life course perspective, with turning points highlighted (for example, 'moving somewhere else', 'new job'); the second stage was based on topics (for example, 'sexual life', 'family relationship', 'healthcare'); and the third stage was based on 'emotional codes' (for example, 'distress', 'happiness', 'enjoyment') associated with each life transition and topic. (For a more detailed discussion of the study methodology and the ethical implications, see Di Feliciantonio, 2021.)

Framing chemsex: sociality, sexual pleasure and the life course

Critical chemsex scholars have highlighted the importance of play and sociality as drivers for chemsex. Drawing from Simmel (1949) and Latour (2005), Race (2015) discusses how the use of the term 'play' within chemsex culture – often referred to as 'party and play' – reveals the central role of sex 'in the assembly of affective associations that Simmel would term "sociability"' (p 259), favouring the formation of a community which is not as stable as the ideal gay community portrayed in most HIV interventions, but '*associated in different forms or assemblages over time*' (p 260, emphasis in original). The interviews realised by Hakim (2019) reveal the sense of togetherness generated by chemsex, as illustrated by the fact that sex itself is only 'one of many group activities that occurred during chemsex sessions, many of which were non-sexual in nature' (p 258), his research participants emphasising the deeply emotional nature of the exchanges occurring during chemsex sessions.

These findings resonate with the narratives of my research participants, the quest for sociality appearing as one of the main reasons to practise chemsex. As explained by Ben, "you hang out, chat, joke, you talk about yourself, ... can be bloody intense but very fun". For Fedex (45–54, Bologna), it is the combination of sex and sociality that drives him towards chemsex: "[Chemsex sessions] have many different moments, it is not just one thing ... what I love the most is going from fucking like an animal to sharing intimate stories in few minutes."

Asked about how chemsex differs from other forms of sociality within the LGBTIQ community in Manchester, Ben's reply questions the overall changes within the gay scene in the city:

'I don't see a community any more. There are many bars, you can see LGBT people everywhere, not just in the Village, but you go there and people are not as friendly as they used to be. Many things have changed. Most of the people I used to hang out [with] left or are dead, ... I have the feeling those places [the bars in the Village] are not for people like me any more.' (Ben)

Fedex's reply to the same question points in a similar direction, even though his narrative seems to focus more on his own life events than on the community around him. Having been in a monogamous relationship for almost a decade, when he broke up with his boyfriend, he found himself "on the market as an HIV-positive over 40 who had forgotten how to hook up and meet new people". This situation made him feel uncomfortable and disconnected; like many other people, he started to use hook-up apps to meet new people, but he was still missing the sense of belonging and sociability that he felt when he was younger and single.

Although framed in a different perspective, both Ben's and Fedex's narratives highlight the interplay between the historical context they live in and individual factors and circumstances that shape people's lives according to the life course approach. Existing scholarship on gay ageing has highlighted the importance of different cultural, social and historical circumstances in shaping the ageing process, such as the central importance attributed to youth and the body in gay culture; the legacy of having gone through the peak of the HIV-AIDS epidemic and the stigma associated with it; and the changing sexual politics of homonormativity (see, for example, Heaphy, 2007; Fredriksen-Goldsen and Muraco, 2010; Lyons et al, 2015; Hammack et al, 2018). However, there is a dimension emerging from the analysis of interviews in my research that has not been adequately discussed in the literature on gay ageing and HIV through a life course perspective: undetectability. What I am arguing here is that to fully understand the practice of chemsex among gay men living with HIV aged over 45, we need to consider how undetectability has represented a sort of game changer in their lives, the perception of their condition and their bodies. In their interviews, all the participants mentioned the importance of undetectability to make them feel better and more at ease with their own bodies.

For Ias (45–54, Manchester), undetectability has given him the opportunity "to play without worrying"; before the advent of undetectability, each sexual encounter carried some sort of negative feeling, making it very difficult for him to relax. "HIV was always in the background somehow", making him paranoid in those situations where there was some exchange of bodily fluids involved, despite him desiring those exchanges. The will to overcome these negative feelings was the original driver for him to start practising sex under the influence of alcohol and/or drugs, well before 'chemsex' was codified and became the object of intense public scrutiny and discussion. In his own words: "it was the only way to relax but also to forget, ... I wanted to bb [bareback] but I was too afraid. Drugs and alcohol were my vehicles to pleasure." The advent of undetectability has somehow reshaped his relationship with sex under influence of drugs.

> 'Now I don't have to forget. I use drugs to enjoy more what I do. Sex is just better with them, but I don't need them as a coping mechanism for my sexual desire [...] I know I cannot transmit the virus to anyone, I don't have to worry about the status of other people [...] it's all about pleasure and having fun.' (Ias)

This improved relationship with his sexual desire has also impacted his approach towards his sexual partners: "In the past I used not to hang out with the same people unless I knew they were poz. ... Now I have several fuck buddies that I have regular fun with. Some of them are negative, but I'm still ok with that." Feeling comfortable with HIV-negative sexual partners seems to relate not just to undetectability, but also to the increasing use of pre-exposure prophylaxis (PrEP) among gay men, especially in the English context. However, most research participants were very sceptical about the real (or, better, fully compliant to guidelines) use of PrEP among chemsex practitioners who claim to be HIV-negative. As discussed by Dree (55–64, London):

> 'I was at some chemsex sessions that lasted two days and I did not see anyone of these young 'negative' guys taking PrEP. ... Personally I think many people are still afraid to say they are positive, but I am in no position to judge, so I don't say anything.' (Dree)

When considering the changing self-perception of one's body as connected to undetectability and chemsex for gay men living with HIV aged over 45, a central dimension that needs to be considered is intergenerationality. In his multi-method study on the life narratives of gays and lesbians aged over 50 in Britain, Heaphy discusses how gay scenes are seen by participants as 'orientated to younger people and explicitly or implicitly ageist' (2009, p 126). For some men, 'gay scenes actively discouraged older people's participation, whilst others noted that they inadequately catered for older people's physical requirements' (Heaphy, 2009, p 126). Participants aged over 45 in my research discuss how chemsex counters ageism within the gay community, bringing together people of different ages. Bonbon (45–54, Manchester) said:

'Guys in their twenties gather with people like me. [...] Not long ago I had a session with a guy who was just 20. We had a really good time. [...] Drugs make you feel comfortable beyond age. [...] I think they really help people who struggle with boundaries, you know?' (Bonbon)

These thoughts are echoed also in the interviews with younger research participants, who discuss how the use of recreational drugs pushes the boundaries of sexual desires beyond what one would 'normally' do. For instance, Sebi (35–44, Milan) described how chemsex allows him not to think about the age and body size of his sexual partners, leading him to question his assumption on the norms behind sexual desire:

'When I'm high, I don't care about your age, I don't care about how big your belly can be, I just enjoy the company of nice people who know how to fuck and want to have a good time. [...] I have come to realise that for most of my life I have completely excluded older, fat men from my sexual imagination. It is like I completely removed them – 'You should not desire those bodies, they are ugly, they are not to have sex with.' [...] Maybe you could say chemsex has taught me something about myself [laughs].' (Sebi)

For some participants, having sexual encounters with younger partners represents the realisation of socially ingrained desires, reinforcing their self-esteem and self-perception. According to Ias:

'There is something [in having sex with younger guys] that you don't get when you have sex with people of your age. [...] I feel more powerful, sexier, hornier. [...] It is what everybody hopes for, isn't it? I mean, many people of my age just pay to have sex with younger guys [...] having them searching [for] me is very, very flattering.' (Ias)

However, intergenerational chemsex encounters also create tensions and ambivalent feelings, especially in the case of very long sessions. As discussed by Ben: "After eight, ten hours I need to stop, I'm just tired. [...] That's the moment when I realise I'm not as young, and that's not a nice feeling." Asked to expand on the feelings experienced in those circumstances, he explained: "probably jealousy first, because I know they're not stopping when I'm stopping, even if they say so. I wish I was younger. Then maybe sadness too, because I'm at home by myself and I wished I could be out there still fucking." Ben's words seem to reproduce the ageist idea that being old is bad because one does not have as much energy as one's younger counterparts (Slevin and Linneman, 2010).

The main strategy developed by participants to feel more integrated with their younger partners in chemsex sessions is over-reliance on sildenafil (or its equivalents) to keep an erection. Most participants mentioned how they always make sure to have it with them before going to any session, while younger participants seem to be less careful in planning their stocks of the drug. However, sildenafil can have heavy side effects, especially if assumed in great quantities. In his interview, Fedex recounted how once he felt he was almost collapsing because he had too much sildenafil. Asked about the reasons behind his choice to take so much of this drug, he explained: "The situation fooled me. I was with these three young guys, very hot. They were all over my cock, so I didn't want to disappoint them. ... It was scary, I really thought I was going to have a heart attack." Asked about the three guys' reaction to the situation, he said: "They were very nice, taking care of me, cuddling me, telling me not to worry. ... But then they invited another top over, because they still wanted to be fucked, so I left." Combined with the other narratives included in this section, Fedex's story highlights the importance of not romanticising chemsex sessions – while they offer the possibility to experiment with sex and sociality, they can also lead to unpleasant experiences that reinforce negative feelings. These ambivalences cannot be separated from different intersections shaping individual experiences, this being the object of the next section.

An intersectional perspective on chemsex

Like any other social phenomenon, the individual experience of chemsex is shaped by the intersection of different axes of social identity. Age and HIV, the main focus of this chapter, intersect with class, race, the performance of masculinity, body shape, among others. Analysis of these intersections exposes different reactions to chemsex among research participants.

Class and economic resources play a very important role: chemsex is based on consumption of (expensive) products, so having enough money to buy them is a prerequisite. Some research participants described the tensions that arise due to the cost of practising chemsex. For instance, Fedex – whose favourite recreational drug is freebase cocaine, costing between €40 and €80 (around £35 to £70) per gram – has spent most of his life savings on buying drugs for chemsex, which makes him feel guilty. In his own words: "When I think about how much I have spent on this, I get so angry with myself ... if tomorrow anything happens to me, I don't have any savings left." These negative feelings seem to be reinforced by intergenerational encounters, as younger sexual partners expect mature men to be wealthier and more generous in buying and sharing drugs. According to Bonbon: "It's hard when you don't have much money to spend on drugs. … The youngsters expect you to pay for the drugs." These thoughts are shared also by younger research participants. Gab (35–44, London) argued: "It's only young guys, especially the hot ones, who might be able not to contribute financially … to be there, older guys have to afford it." However, the same tensions do not emerge in the narratives of wealthier research participants. For example, Ias, who has a well-paid job, explained that he does not mind buying drugs for everyone: "It's just about having a good time. It doesn't matter how much it is."

Strictly related to economic resources and class, homeownership, or, more generally, having an autonomous living situation, influences the experience of chemsex as well. In Ben's opinion: "When you own your house, you don't have to worry too much about other people – you can have ten guys over." Having a big house seems to play a very favourable role, especially in very expensive locations such as London and Milan. In contrast, people who live in social housing and/or share the house they live in with someone else described a more difficult situation, having to rely on others hosting chemsex sessions. In Bonbon's words: "It would be nice to have people over whenever I want, but I have to make sure they [the people he lives with] are not there. … It requires a lot of planning."

Race also seems to play an ambivalent role in the narratives of non-White participants. For instance, Bonbon (who identifies as Black) explained how being Black allows him to receive many more invitations from younger guys than other men of his age, even though he cannot always afford to buy the drugs. In his opinion, this stems from the widespread fantasy of Black guys having bigger penises and being more wild (Lemelle, 2010). However, this process of sexual racialisation also causes uncomfortable situations, notably when sexual partners push him to embody their 'Black man fantasy' and/or they express disappointment in his failure/refusal to embody their requests. For instance, he explained that when he joins a group at someone's place, "they want me to top straight away. … Sometimes it's fun, because I want it, but sometimes I wanna bottom first or I don't get hard and people come with nasty racist jokes." Similar experiences are narrated by other non-White research participants.

Other important axes of identity that shape the experience of chemsex are the performance of masculinity and body size. This is highlighted clearly in the following statement by Dree: "These young guys wanna live the daddy fantasy. You can't be femme, they want you strong and masculine." This statement is in line with well-established academic arguments on hegemonic masculinities within gay communities (for example, Phua, 2002). This process does not seem to be really challenged in chemsex sessions, as confirmed also by the narratives of younger research participants. For example, Tariq (25–34, Milan) framed his sexual desire for older men during chemsex sessions as driven by the fantasy of being "dominated. [...] You want your daddy to be virile and strong, you don't want him to be a queen." This quest for older guys who embody a hegemonic masculinity can provoke tensions and discomfort among older participants. According to Ias: "There is a limit. I'm up for playing the master daddy fantasy, but at the end of the day I'm there to have a good time and be relaxed. I don't want the pressure of wondering 'am I being masc enough?'" Body size appears to be strictly related to the performance of masculinity. Men with big bodies (not necessarily heavily muscled) were usually described as more sexually attractive. This is reflected in the following quote by Green Eyes (18–24, Manchester): "Big older guys are sexy, I want them to dom me. [...] It is weird when there is an older guy who's short, slim or bottom only. [...] It's not the kind of fantasy I have." Taken together, these quotes reveal the persistence of hegemonic ideals about the body and masculinity within gay communities, even in situations of sexual experimentation.

Conclusion

In recent years, chemsex has become the object of intense public scrutiny, mainly based on pathologising and panic-raising narratives. Rejecting the assumptions of most public health-inspired academic analyses of chemsex, scholars across the social sciences and cultural studies have started to produce a critical, historical and social conceptualisation of this phenomenon. Despite the effort to expand the breath of chemsex studies in order to include more subjectivities, the relationship between some markers of identity and chemsex remains understudied – age(ing) being one of them. Building on the narratives of gay men living with HIV in England and Italy, this chapter has shown how age(ing) shapes an ambivalent relationship with chemsex. Echoing previous analyses (for example, Hakim, 2019), research participants emphasise how chemsex favours new forms of sociality and sexual pleasure, made possible also by the advent of the paradigm of undetectability, which makes them feel more comfortable with their own bodies. However, the adoption of an intergenerational and intersectional perspective complicates their narratives: chemsex can also create uncomfortable situations and negative feelings, while also reproducing unequal social relations along the lines of, among others, age, class, race, performance of masculinity and body size. These findings caution against the impulse to romanticise chemsex as some form of new utopic reality that can overcome social inequalities, while also considering its radical potential in terms of sexual pleasure and unexpected social encounters.

The analysis developed in the chapter presents clear limitations, the main one being the age of the participants. None were over the age of 65. In most research, the participants would be identified as being in 'midlife' (Simpson,

2013), even though HIV-related research (problematically) still considers 50 the threshold for 'ageing' for people living with HIV. While the difficulties of recruiting participants aged over 65 can be connected to the dramatic impact of HIV/AIDS on the life expectancy of gay male baby boomers across the Minority World (Rosenfeld et al, 2012), we can now expect an increasing number of people living with HIV who will live well beyond 65 thanks to advances in biomedical technologies and access to ART. We know little about the relationship between sexual practices, drugs (both licit and illicit) and the uncertainty provoked by ageing with HIV; grounded, empirical research is therefore needed to start filling this wide gap in knowledge. This effort has the potential to make chemsex research more inclusive of specific age groups and sexual practices (see, for instance, Sandberg, 2019, on the sexualisation of touch for ageing men, destabilising the centrality assigned to the sexual phallic male body), while also making social science HIV research more attentive to the dimensions of pleasure and desire.

Acknowledgements
This research was supported by the European Commission, MSCA-IF-EF-ST Action, grant number 747110.

References
Bourne, A., Reid, D., Hickson, F., Torres-Rueda, S. and Weatherburn, P. (2015) 'Illicit drug use in sexual settings ("chemsex") and HIV/STI transmission risk behaviour among gay men in South London: findings from a qualitative study', *Sexually Transmitted Infections*, 91(8): 564–8.

Brennan, D.J., Hellerstedt, W.L., Ross, M.W. and Welles, S.L. (2007) 'History of childhood sexual abuse and HIV risk behaviors in homosexual and bisexual men', *American Journal of Public Health*, 97(6): 1107–12.

Brotman, S., Silverman, M., Boska, H. and Molgat, M. (2020) 'Intergenerational care in the context of migration: a feminist intersectional life-course exploration of racialized young adult women's narratives of care', *Affilia* [online]. doi: 10.1177/0886109920954408.

Brown, G. and Di Feliciantonio, C. (2022) 'Geographies of PrEP, TasP and undetectability: reconceptualising HIV assemblages to explore what else matters in the lives of gay and bisexual men', *Dialogues in Human Geography*, 12(1): 100–18.

Brown, M. (2012) 'Gender and sexuality I: Intersectional anxieties', *Progress in Human Geography*, 36(4): 541–50.

Bryant, J., Hopwood, M., Dowsett, G.W., Aggleton, P., Holt, M., Lea, T., Drysdale, K. and Treloar, C. (2018) 'The rush to risk when interrogating the relationship between methamphetamine use and sexual practice among gay and bisexual men', *International Journal of Drug Policy*, 55: 242–8.

Chapman, E. (2000) 'Conceptualisation of the body for people living with HIV: issues of touch and contamination', *Sociology of Health & Illness*, 22(6): 840–57.

Collins, P.H. and Bilge, S. (2016) *Intersectionality*, Cambridge: Policy Press.

Crenshaw, K. (1991) 'Mapping the margins', *Stanford Law Review*, 43: 1241–99.

Davis, K. (2008) 'Intersectionality as buzzword: a sociology of science perspective on what makes a feminist theory successful', *Feminist Theory*, 9(1): 67–85.

Dennis, F. (2019) *Injecting Bodies in More-than-Human Worlds*, London: Routledge.

Dhamoon, R. (2011) 'Considerations on mainstreaming intersectionality', *Political Research Quarterly*, 64(1): 230–43.

Di Feliciantonio, C. (2021) '(Un)ethical boundaries: critical reflections on what we are (not) supposed to do', *The Professional Geographer*, 73(3): 496–503.

Drysdale, K. (2021) '"Scene" as a critical framing device: extending analysis of chemsex cultures', *Sexualities* [online]. doi: 10.1177/1363460721995467

Drysdale, K., Bryant, J., Hopwood, M., Dowsett, G.W., Holt, M., Lea, T., Aggleton, P. and Treloar, C. (2020) 'Destabilising the "problem" of chemsex: diversity in settings, relations and practices revealed in Australian gay and bisexual men's crystal methamphetamine use', *International Journal of Drug Policy* [online], 78: 102697. doi: 10.1016/j.drugpo.2020.102697

Elder, G.H., Jr (1994) 'Time, human agency, and social change: perspectives on the life course', *Social Psychology Quarterly*, 57(1): 4–15.

Ferrer, I., Grenier, A., Brotman, S. and Koehn, S. (2017) 'Understanding the experiences of racialized older people through an intersectional life course perspective', *Journal of Aging Studies*, 41: 10–17.

Florêncio, J. (2021) 'Chemsex cultures: subcultural reproduction and queer survival', *Sexualities* [online]. doi: 10.1177/1363460720986922.

Fredriksen-Goldsen, K.I. and Muraco, A. (2010) 'Aging and sexual orientation: a 25-year review of the literature', *Research on Aging*, 32(3): 372–413.

Hagestad, G.O. and Uhlenberg, P. (2005) 'The social separation of old and young: a root of ageism', *Journal of Social Issues*, 61(2): 343–60.

Hakim, J. (2019) 'The rise of chemsex: queering collective intimacy in neoliberal London', *Cultural Studies*, 33(2): 249–75.

Halberstam, J. (2005) *In a Queer Time and Place: Transgender Bodies, Subcultural Lives*, New York: New York University Press.

Hammack, P.L., Frost, D.M., Meyer, I.H. and Pletta, D.R. (2018) 'Gay men's health and identity: social change and the life course', *Archives of Sexual Behavior*, 47(1): 59–74.

Heaphy, B. (2007) 'Sexualities, gender and ageing: resources and social change', *Current Sociology*, 55(2): 193–210.

Heaphy, B. (2009) 'Choice and its limits in older lesbian and gay narratives of relational life', *Journal of GLBT Family Studies*, 5(1–2): 119–38.

Heidari, S. (2016) 'Sexuality and older people: a neglected issue', *Reproductive Health Matters*, 24(48): 1–5.

Hopkins, P. (2019) 'Social geography I: intersectionality', *Progress in Human Geography*, 43(5): 937–47.

Hopkins, P. and Pain, R. (2007) 'Geographies of age: thinking relationally', *Area*, 39(3): 287–94.

Kirby, T. and Thornbur-Dunwell, M. (2013) 'High-risk drug practices tighten grip on London gay scene', *The Lancet*, 381(9861): 101–2.

Latour, B. (2005) *Reassembling the Social: An Introduction to Actor-Network Theory*, Oxford: Oxford University Press.

Lemelle, A.J., Jr (2010) *Black Masculinity and Sexual Politics*, New York: Routledge.

Lovelock, M. (2018) 'Sex, death and austerity: resurgent homophobia in the British tabloid press', *Critical Studies in Media Communication*, 35(3): 225–39.

Lyons, A., Croy, S., Barrett, C. and Whyte, C. (2015) 'Growing old as a gay man: how life has changed for the gay liberation generation', *Ageing & Society*, 35(10): 2229–50.

Mayer, K.U. (2009) 'New directions in life course research', *Annual Review of Sociology*, 35: 413–33.

Mojola, S.A., Williams, J., Angotti, N. and Gómez-Olivé, F.X. (2015) 'HIV after 40 in rural South Africa: a life course approach to HIV vulnerability among middle aged and older adults', *Social Science & Medicine*, 143: 204–12.

Møller, K. and Hakim, J. (2021) 'Critical chemsex studies: interrogating cultures of sexualized drug use beyond the risk paradigm', *Sexualities* [online]. doi: 10.1177/13634607211026223.

Nash, J.C. (2008) 'Re-thinking intersectionality', *Feminist Review*, 89(1): 1–15.

Phua, V.C. (2002) 'Sex and sexuality in men's personal advertisements', *Men and Masculinities*, 5(2): 178–91.

Pienaar, K., Murphy, D.A., Race, K. and Lea, T. (2020) 'Drugs as technologies of the self: enhancement and transformation in LGBTQ cultures', *International Journal of Drug Policy* [online], 78: 102673. doi: 10.1016/j.drugpo.2020.102673

Race, K. (2015) '"Party and play": online hook-up devices and the emergence of PNP practices among gay men', *Sexualities*, 18(3): 253–75.

Race, K. (2018) *The Gay Science: Intimate Experiments with the Problem of HIV*, London: Routledge.

Rosenfeld, D., Bartlam, B. and Smith, R.D. (2012) 'Out of the closet and into the trenches: gay male baby boomers, aging, and HIV/AIDS', *The Gerontologist*, 52(2): 255–64.

Ruark, A., Kennedy, C.E., Mazibuko, N., Dlamini, L., Nunn, A., Green, E.C. and Surkan, P.J. (2016) 'From first love to marriage and maturity: a life-course perspective on HIV risk among young Swazi adults', *Culture, Health & Sexuality*, 18(7): 812–25.

Sandberg, L.J. (2019) 'Closer to touch: sexuality, embodiment and masculinity in older men's lives', in S. Katz (ed) *Ageing in Everyday Life*, Bristol: Policy Press, pp 129–44.

Settersten, R.A. and Mayer, K.U. (1997) 'The measurement of age, age structuring, and the life course', *Annual Review of Sociology*, 23: 233–61.

Simmel, G. (1949) 'The sociology of sociability', *American Journal of Sociology*, 55(3): 254–61.

Simpson, P. (2013) 'Alienation, ambivalence, agency: middle-aged gay men and ageism in Manchester's gay village', *Sexualities*, 16(3–4): 283–99.

Simpson, P. (2014) 'Differentiating selves: middle-aged gay men in Manchester's less visible "homospaces"', *The British Journal of Sociology*, 65(1): 150–69.

Slevin, K.F. and Linneman, T.J. (2010) 'Old gay men's bodies and masculinities', *Men and Masculinities*, 12(4): 483–507.

Stuart, D. (2013) 'Sexualised drug use by MSM: background, current status and response', *HIV Nursing*, 13(1): 6–10.

Tester, G. (2018) '"And then AIDS came along": a life course turning point and sub-cohorts of older gay men', *Journal of Gay & Lesbian Social Services*, 30(1): 33–48.

Vanderbeck, R. (2007) 'Intergenerational geographies: age relations, segregation and reengagements', *Geography Compass*, 1(2): 200–21.

Walker, L. (2020) 'Problematising the discourse of "post-AIDS"', *Journal of Medical Humanities*, 41(2): 95–105.

Wengraf, T. (2001) *Qualitative Research Interviewing: Biographic Narrative and Semi-Structured Methods*, London: Sage.

5

Freed from fear: reconstructing older gay male sexuality through PrEP – an account of a generational experience

Jacek Kolodziej

Introduction

The generational trauma of the AIDS crisis profoundly impacted the ways in which gay men coming of age at the time of the epidemic engaged in sexual practices and connected with one another. In this chapter, I propose a way to reconstruct the impacts of novel methods of prevention that change the perceptions of HIV prevention and sexual practices among gay men in later life who had experienced the trauma of the AIDS crisis first-hand. I present an account of Allan (pseudonym), a gay man in his sixties, as a case of recovering the joy and intimacy of sexual encounters among those whose lives had been deeply affected by the catastrophic generational experience. In focusing on the account of a single gay man, I intend to contextualise his experience within the trajectory of his life and – as Allan understood it – the story of his generation.

In the first section of this chapter, I present a generational approach to social HIV research, including some of the most commonly used age cohort classifications. In the sections that follow, I introduce Allan and present his account, highlighting the reconstruction of his understandings of AIDS history as he begins using biomedical HIV prevention. In this chapter, I focus on the aspects of gay HIV experience that are common for many Western countries with low-level epidemics concentrated in gay and bisexual communities. This is despite the fact that the experience of the AIDS crisis in Aotearoa New Zealand was in many ways unique; interested readers may find it described in detail in the works of other authors (for example, Davis, 1996, Dickson et al, 2015). In particular, the existing research contains rich accounts of the experiences of HIV by Aotearoa New Zealand's Indigenous people, the Māori (see, for instance, Grierson et al, 2004; Henrickson, 2006; Aspin, 2007; Rua'ine, 2007).

The method of HIV prevention at the centre of this chapter is pre-exposure prophylaxis (PrEP). This involves taking antiretroviral medication prior to sexual HIV exposure in order to reduce the risk of HIV acquisition. The effectiveness of PrEP alone is so high that on a practical level, when used correctly, it virtually removes the risk of HIV for its users (BPAC NZ, 2019). Despite the fact that PrEP does not reduce the risk of contracting other sexually transmitted infections (STIs), a number of PrEP users may opt not to use condoms, as infections other than HIV are typically associated with less perceived social and medical burden (Wells, 2020).

Generational approach

Before I introduce Allan's account, and by way of background to this chapter, I signal some general historical developments relevant for many Western countries. PrEP emerged in the social setting of the aftermath from the AIDS crisis and its trauma. In the early 1980s, AIDS seemed to have appeared out of nowhere and spread rapidly through the communities first deemed high risk. At the time, AIDS equalled death, and there were no effective treatments to help those diagnosed (Shilts, 1988). However, meaningful community responses and almost unprecedented medical advances led to spectacular leaps in treatment and profound improvements in outcomes (Palella et al, 1998) within just two decades. In other words, men born in the mid-1960s or earlier witnessed distinctly different eras of sexual safety and enacting same-sex desire. First, there was the pre-AIDS era, when condoms were used only to prevent unwanted pregnancy among heterosexual couples and there were no apparent mortal health threats associated with same-sex practices. Second, there was a sudden emergence of an unexpected, deadly and quickly spreading disease that caused deaths of a significant number of gay men. This resulted in the naturalisation of the imperative to reduce sexual activity and use condoms to evade the existential threat and preserve life.[1]

The advent of zidovudine (also known as AZT) in the 1980s demonstrated that, maybe, HIV infection did not have to be deadly. In the 1990s, a significant treatment advancement – the development of protease inhibitors and highly active antiretroviral therapy – marked the time when HIV infection started to transform into a chronic illness that would not lead inevitably to death. These changes were associated with profound impacts on those affected, with some referring to the effects of new treatments as

---

[1] This is of course a simplified summary. It should be noted that discrimination, along with medical inequities (and activism), was present among gay communities before the AIDS crisis; this has been documented in literature (Batza, 2018). Also, the reconstructions of the history of gay desire post AIDS have been contested, and the detrimental consequences of AIDS discourses for the sexual cultures of gay men have been discussed (Rofes, 1998).

the 'Lazarus syndrome' when describing the experiences of those who had reconciled with imminent death only later to discover that they would live (Brashers et al, 1999). The two most recent decades were characterised by gradual improvement in therapies and in the quality of life of people living with HIV who could access one of many available treatments, though face persisting social stigma. Despite the advancements, HIV continues to have deadly sequelae for those with severely delayed diagnosis or poor access to medical treatment. The emergence of conclusive evidence that virally suppressed individuals cannot transmit HIV sexually (undetectable equals untransmittable: U=U) marked a significant milestone both for HIV prevention and in the context of combatting HIV stigma (Prevention Access Campaign, 2016).

The social effects of HIV were so significant that it has been proposed that they led to a differentiation of specific generational identities in gay men (Halkitis, 2014, 2019; Gardiner, 2018; Hammack et al, 2018; Bower et al, 2019). The theoretical assumptions underpinning the generational analysis stem primarily from life course theory (Elder et al, 2003). In order to define the *generation* (the term often used interchangeably with *cohort*), it is necessary to identify important *cohort-defining events* that occur during the *critical periods*, typically puberty and emerging adulthood (Hammack et al, 2018). Various attempts have been made to define these critical events and their associated generations, and for many cohorts of gay men they centre around gay rights and HIV. Of course, within a given generation, diverse personal beliefs and reactions may develop in response to the critical events, and the extent to which individuals are affected may vary greatly. In this way, life course theory emphasises intra-generational similarities and intergenerational differences while paying less attention to individual differences (Elder et al, 2003).

In order to put Allan's experience in context, it is useful to consider the generational division theory developed by Hammack et al (2018). This relies on the concept of cohort-defining events, with a strong emphasis on the impacts of AIDS. The authors distinguished five cohorts, labelling them by referencing the critical notions contemporary to the time of coming of age. These generations are: the Sickness Generation – born in the 1930s, they came of age when same-sex desire was classified as an illness; the Liberation Generation – born in the 1940s, they experienced early adulthood when the gay rights movement was gaining momentum, and their social and romantic networks were strongly impacted by AIDS; the AIDS-1 Generation – born in the 1950s and 1960s, they experienced early adulthood at the height of the AIDS crisis and experienced loss of friends and lovers; the AIDS-2 Generation – born in 1970s and 1980s, they experienced fewer personal losses due to AIDS, but gay sex was equated with death; and the Equality Generation – born in the 1990s, they experienced significant advancements in recognition and acceptance of gay men, along with establishment of effective HIV treatments.[2]

While these generational classifications have been defined within the US context, the cohort-defining moments are not unique to the American experience, though other important events could be more relevant locally. In many British Commonwealth countries, when attempting periodisation of gay rights advancements, many legal and cultural frames of reference are situated in the United Kingdom. An important milestone in law reform both in the United Kingdom and, later, in Aotearoa New Zealand (Bennett, 2009) was the release of the 1957 *Report of the Departmental Committee on Homosexual Offences and Prostitution* (Cmnd 267; better known as the Wolfenden Report), which called for decriminalisation of consensual and private homosexual activity. The report influenced the legal systems in many Commonwealth jurisdictions.[3] The recommendations from the report were, however, implemented at different paces in different countries (Kirby, 2008), with England and Wales decriminalising homosexuality first in 1967, a decade after the report was published.

The New Zealand Homosexual Law Reform Act 1986 and its preceding community activism encouraged by legal changes in other countries following the release of the Wolfenden Report (Bennett, 2009) were likely a cohort-defining moment in Aotearoa New Zealand. The legal and political changes brought by the Act coincided with the trauma of AIDS. Importantly, the community organisations that were first created to advocate for the rights of gay men, such as the National Gay Rights Coalition, or community outlets dedicated to gay rights, like *Pink Triangle*, provided the first social response and focused on the issues of HIV prevention (Lindberg and McMorland, 1996). The National Gay Rights Coalition, which had discontinued activity in 1981, was reactivated in 1983 specifically to provide advocacy and community support and education around HIV/ AIDS (Parkinson and Hughes, 1987). The struggle to end discriminatory laws coincided with the early emergence of HIV. In this chapter, I use the term 'AIDS generation' to denote a cohort of men born in Aotearoa New Zealand in the 1950s and 1960s, underlining the important cumulative social

---

[2] Comparison of responses to PrEP in the AIDS-1 Generation and younger cohorts does not present a clear-cut picture. In an American study of views on PrEP, older men – contrary to some opinions about this group's conservativeness – tended to share positive views with the youngest generations, emphasising the HIV spread-control benefits of PrEP. However, they showed lower levels of appreciation than younger groups for PrEP's anxiety-reducing and sex-enhancing qualities (Hammack et al, 2019).

[3] Despite significant progress in many jurisdictions, as of 2021, 36 out of 53 Commonwealth countries continued to criminalise homosexuality (BBC, 2021).

effects of the decriminalisation and AIDS activism movements among men reaching their early adulthood in the 1980s.

Meeting Allan

To illustrate the reconstruction of AIDS history as informed by the emergence of novel methods of prevention, I present the story of Allan, a member of the AIDS generation. When we first met, Allan was a gay man in his sixties who identified as a New Zealand European (known as 'White' or 'Caucasian' in other contexts) and was professionally active in a skilled occupation. He wanted to share his story about PrEP use to benefit others who might use it. At the time of our interviews, Allan lived in a long-term open relationship with his partner, who, by Allan's account, was also using PrEP. Allan had started using PrEP around 12 months before the first interview took place.

As part of a larger project (approved by Massey University Human Ethics Committee; NOR 17/43), I interviewed Allan twice. To elicit deeply contextual reconstruction, a Gadamerian interviewing method was used; this focuses on the participant's own understandings of the topics discussed. It is important to note that Gadamerian epistemology emphasises the intersubjective nature of meaning construction and truth, their historicity, and reliance on pre-understandings (prejudices) of the dialogue participants, as opposed to trying to suspend one's own judgments in an attempt to uncover 'objective' truths (Gadamer, 1975; Laverty, 2003; Debesay et al, 2008; Paul, 2012). The interview topics included HIV prevention and sexual practices. The interviews were audio-recorded and transcribed verbatim for analyses that employed an abductive process (Brinkmann, 2014) and Gadamerian principles of interpretation. These include the hermeneutic circle (circular analysis: whole-to-parts and parts-to-whole), consideration of historicity (here, the changing contexts of social functioning of gay men and HIV prevention), and fusion of horizons (engaging with one's own pre-understandings of the phenomena in question).

Generational breakthroughs

The trauma of the AIDS crisis affected the men of Allan's age cohort, the AIDS generation, profoundly. When I interviewed Allan, I understood that as I was roughly half his age and had not personally experienced the AIDS crisis in the same way he did, my ideas of radical change in the well-being of gay communities following changes in HIV prevention might be vastly different from his. I shared my thinking with Allan to try to understand if and how he perceived a radical change brought about by PrEP:

Jacek: I obviously come from a different generation ... I can't even fathom the pre-AIDS era, when you didn't think about condoms. ... I can't relate personally to that experience of [the] pre-AIDS era, but you've obviously been through that era and then through the worst of AIDS. So, do you think PrEP is such a milestone here?

Allan: I think it's a huge milestone. I think PrEP in conjunction with U=U, I think they're both huge milestones. They're both complete game changers.

Allan shared the view that PrEP was a "game changer" for gay communities and HIV prevention. He added that this was the case for the two new effective biomedical interventions: PrEP and the knowledge that undetectable viral load stops ongoing HIV transmission (U=U).

Allan felt that the broader history of HIV aligned with the trajectory of his sexual life. PrEP shaped the dramatic shifts in his prevention practices as he aged and felt increasingly emotionally mature.

> '[Time on PrEP] has been incredible, very much so. I think it's just because when I first came out, condoms were for preventing pregnancy. So, I'm not making anyone pregnant, and then, what now seems to be almost overnight, the whole behaviour is changing and just having to go through decades just being very cautious and very considered about what I'm doing, then suddenly going on a pill. Not only has it flipped right back again, but it's flipped back again at a time when I'm older! I'm probably a lot more confident than I was when I was younger, just an age-related thing, different world view, different attitude to people, and behaviour, that's the thing. I'm feeling now that when I was younger, I tended to [be a] relatively cautious person. But people who enjoyed themselves more are dead. I just feel in some ways very lucky, but now I can enjoy myself. I'm [in my sixties], I'm not 22, and I can enjoy myself without having to worry [about] sort of going through ... and to lose that again would be very, very difficult.' (Allan)

The changes he experienced were truly transformative, and Allan was grateful for them. He felt that because he went through decades of caution and fear, he was prepared to appreciate the changes brought on by PrEP that restored some aspects of the pre-AIDS era and, in a way, brought him a second youth. Allan felt that he had survived the advent of the epidemic because he had been so cautious in his youth, while others, perhaps more sexually adventurous men, had not. Allan also believed that as he had matured emotionally and become more confident, PrEP was even more appropriate for the older version of himself, as he could appreciate it more.

Trauma and disbelief

Allan's story clearly illustrates the changing social landscapes of the early 1980s, as the early AIDS activism he was involved in had evolved naturally from his earlier participation in the gay rights movement. Allan shared how the AIDS crisis impacted on his young adulthood.

'I think I mentioned to you, in my twenties I had my first overseas trip and I followed the gay man's sort of holiday. I went to San Francisco, New York, and just two or three months before I left, the first news of AIDS, headlines of Kaposi's sarcoma. I just didn't want to know! I was going on holiday, and I was going to have fun ... I went and ... I knew absolutely nothing. I was involved quite politically at the time, with the [named gay organisation]. ... When the first news started coming out of San Francisco in 1981, we heard that, I heard it. It was just, we didn't know what to make of it. Gay men started to die of Kaposi's sarcoma, it wasn't known why or how. I was going on my big holiday overseas! I was going to the hotspots and I was going to have fun, and nothing was going to stop me. And I had fun. I wasn't going to have a baby, so why use condoms? When I got back then, I came back with gonorrhoea and was ... getting more information coming through. Then it really hit me, just really sank in. I thought, "holy shit". As soon as the test, it took time, but when tests became available, I had a test as soon as they were available, incredibly relieved to find I was negative. But at that stage people [were] starting to come down with HIV, come down with being really sick and I started to, you were at the stage when someone went into hospital, with just that isolation! Wave at them through a glass, with a note, that sort of thing. People just disappeared! They'd start getting sick and then they go back to where they live, go back to family, and [you] never hear or see them again. ... Most ended up going back to their families and their families just closed around, shut up, because it's such a shameful thing. Isolated them and we'd find out later they'd died. ... Yes, I was incredibly lucky, so I just became, I suppose, in a way, quite evangelical about using condoms [and] doing what I could to spread the safe sex message.' (Allan)

Through this powerful account, Allan positioned HIV prevention in the context of his life course as superimposed on the historic trajectory of AIDS over the last few decades. He realised he had been at heightened risk when no preventive measures were known or used, and he considered himself lucky to have survived through this period. At the time, he believed his risk was extremely high; in the 1980s, an HIV diagnosis effectively meant a death sentence for many. His first HIV test was a source of distress, followed by unexpected relief when the result came back as negative. He witnessed first-hand people he had known dying in shame and isolation, and this trauma led him to use condoms religiously as well as to become an avid supporter of "the safe sex message". This generation-defining experience informed Allan's sexual health choices for decades to come and bound condom use with the notion of survival.

For Allan, the experience of radical change centred around freeing himself from the feelings of shame and guilt that arose over the years and were rooted in the generational experience of the AIDS crisis.

> 'I read a couple of reports, mainly from North America, of gay men similar age to me who had been through the worst of the AIDS crisis, come out the other end. Completely, totally unexpected reaction of going on PrEP and suddenly peeling away, very quickly, peeling away all these layers of caution, shame, guilt. Just be able, I don't know any other way of describing [the] absolute joy of pleasure, of just being able to enjoy other men.' (Allan)

Starting PrEP had a profound emotional impact on Allan, and that was not something he had been expecting. When he read accounts from the United States of other PrEP users of similar age and with personal biographies quite like his, the similarity of their experiences resonated strongly with him. In the quote above, Allan recounted all the feelings that had become attached to expressing himself sexually, which PrEP has now removed: caution, guilt, and shame. The process of disassociating sexuality from these strong negative connotations was cathartic. For Allan, PrEP was an agent of transformation that replaced the difficult emotions with pure joy, pleasure and feelings of connectedness to other men. Allan's metaphor of peeling away the layers suggests that these emotions were in fact a residue of living with fear of HIV that was distorting his connections with other men and genuine sexual experience.

> 'It's almost like pinching myself at times. ... Just something that just wouldn't and couldn't happen 12 months ago, or 18 months ago. It's not only the perspective of condoms, it's the whole, it's the thing that I wasn't expecting. It was the whole emotional change of how [I have] emotionally adapted to being safe and being cautious, and it influenced and pervaded just being intimate with people.' (Allan)

Only through the removal of strong negative feelings associated with connecting with other men was Allan able to fully recognise the extent to which fear of HIV had impacted his relationships and his quality of life. He recounted how unexpected the emotional transformation owing to

PrEP had been for him. From this new perspective, Allan was able to see that many decades of caution caused by fear of HIV had diminished his ability to become intimate with other men. Gay men have formed unique cultural practices around expressing, sharing and manifesting sexuality. These were strongly affected, if not transformed, by the biological reality and threat of AIDS, which resulted in radical changes in sexual practices (Crossley, 2004), activism and advocacy (Altman, 2013; Hindman, 2019), and identity formation (Grierson and Smith, 2005). Allan witnessed many of these changes first-hand. Importantly, he clearly remembered the time when condoms were not commonly used by gay men, as there were no known life-threatening STIs.

Community connection

Allan's story shows how important experiencing sex was in his life. Other than being simply an enjoyable experience, sex with other men was, for him, a way of seeking connectedness with others:

> 'Even anonymously ... like in a sex club with someone I've never met before, if they're having a good time and seem to be enjoying themselves and I'm enjoying myself, we may only be together a half an hour ... I think it's a much better social communication than many other forms of social communication.' (Allan)

Allan understood engaging in sex, even with anonymous partners, as a meaningful way to communicate with his fellow men. Sharing pleasure was an important way of connecting that could even be superior to many other forms of social communication, as it involved opening up to other humans and reflecting one another's emotional and sensual states. The transformative potential of PrEP allowed this process of connecting to unfold uninterrupted, but it is worth noting that for Allan, condomless sex was not a goal in itself, but rather a means to enhance intimacy.

It has been argued that the AIDS crisis effectively desexed the gay liberation movement and its culture in the West (Hindman, 2019). The prevailing narrative informs that the emergence of a serious biological threat and the menace of the early epidemic creeping out of its initial gay pockets put pressure on the gay movements to restrain the march towards greater sexual liberation and start self-policing the dangerous sexual practices of its members (Hindman, 2019). The perfect storm for these processes to develop occurred in connection with the wider phenomenon of a largely consumerist drive to normative social participation (Duggan, 2002) and de-queering in order to be granted a place at the table (Bawer, 1993) in the mainstream political landscape.

The sanitisation of gay practices and bodies within the gay communities may be a response to their earlier biological and symbolic contamination by HIV.[4] Allan's story reflects these narratives clearly, as he spoke about the mistrust, fear and reservations he had been experiencing prior to the use of PrEP. In his account, PrEP purified the male body, which was no longer seen as a threat, but rather as an object of desire and a source of pleasure. It has been robustly theorised (Holmes and Warner, 2005; Dean, 2009; Garcia, 2013) that the allure of bareback sex (as opposed to bug chasing, actively seeking to acquire HIV) lies not in the possibility of contamination, but in fantasies about insemination, creation, reproduction and connection through symbolic kinship. Now, with PrEP, these fantasies could be successfully, and more safely, recovered for those who remember the pre-AIDS era.

Shame and internalised guilt

Allan had never experienced any form of stigmatisation associated with his PrEP use, though he had expected that to happen.

'I haven't personally experienced it [shaming for the use of PrEP]. I'm sure it must exist here. I wonder if it's perhaps less of an issue here. I think probably [it] is less of an issue. I have seen a couple of online comments in New Zealand where I've thought it's probably more [of] a matter of education rather than anything else. Nothing serious.' (Allan)

Despite not having experienced slut shaming (stigma associated with sexual activity perceived as excessive) himself, Allan strongly suspected there was an undercurrent of prejudiced attitudes in the gay communities. The lack of first-hand experience of these attitudes led Allan to question why he had such a strong expectation that he would experience slut shaming.

'I had wondered, I sometimes wonder if it's my fear of slut shaming that mostly has led to an expectation to be so, who knows ... I don't know, I wonder if it's my sort of feelings about sex. Because I sometimes have Calvinistic thoughts as well, that I have to sort of rationalise. Is it just ... [the] Calvinist in me sort of saying, "You're just a dirty slut, shame on you"? ... For me, I wonder if it's more an echo of the past decades of ... "I must use condoms all the time"'. (Allan)

---

[4] The proliferation in the gay community of the term 'clean' to denote HIV-negative individuals, with its implicit antonym of 'dirty', provides a linguistic key that helps make sense of the symbolic representations of HIV.

Allan felt that his expectations of anti-PrEP sentiment in the community may have stemmed from his internalised shame and reservations about sexuality. Calling his thoughts "Calvinistic", he referred to the strict, conservative mores that largely reject sexuality, especially pleasure-oriented sexuality. He recounted his internal moral struggle ("You're just a dirty slut, shame on you") around the ethics of sexual expression, which he linked to the newer homonormative notions of good and responsible homosexual men that should shy away from condom non-use. There is a broader context with similar experiences, suggesting a more universal characteristic of this gay experience. To quote Rofes (1998, p 157), 'I believe increasing evidence that many gay men occasionally fuck without condoms taps into an immense pool of sexual shame long lurking just under the surface of gay men's communities.'

The changing of social norms, informed by the implicit disposition that emphasises a sex-positive approach, influenced Allan's sexual practices: "[I don't use condoms now] unless someone else specifically asks for them. ... Sex is about sharing pleasure and sharing intimacy. If someone else is going to feel uncomfortable about their safety, that's not sharing." Allan made it clear that his choice not to use condoms was to allow greater intimacy with his sexual partners. However, he was ready to use condoms if his partners needed them to feel safe and comfortable when having sex. He recognised that condomless sex while using PrEP was what provided him with the feeling of safety but for others, that same comfort could only be achieved through sex with condoms. In other words, Allan valued the connection afforded by sexual contact with other men when both partners felt safe and comfortable, and the choice of method of prevention served that greater goal of intimacy.

Crossley (2004) argues that the notions of 'resistance' and 'transgression' have formed an important part of gay men's social habitus[5] since the early days of the liberation movement. Crossley (2007) argues that these embodied dispositions of gay men are intrinsically connected to the notions of transgression, resistance and liberation through sexuality. Rofes (1998) elaborates why gay men with good knowledge of HIV/AIDS engage, at times, in some riskier sex practices as a resistance to mainstream social norms:

Many gay men consider sex to be an activity of central value to our identities and lives. We may see it as a survival strategy that makes living satisfying and worthwhile. This does not mean we are obsessed with

---

[5] Here, the author refers to Bourdieu's (1977) notion of habitus, emphasising the subconscious embodied dispositions that govern making sense of the world and the social practices of individuals and larger social units.

sex or have no interests or activities besides sex. It means we value the enactment of our desires and will not always give them up in a grand gesture of sacrifice to the epidemic. (Rofes, 1998, p 225)

Mending the broken community

Another source of the feelings of guilt Allan experienced prior to PrEP was serosorting (purposeful selection of partners of the same HIV status), which he sometimes employed as a supplementary method of HIV prevention.

Because of his earlier personal losses, along with witnessing profound isolation of HIV-positive members of his community in the early days of the AIDS crisis, he considered avoiding people living with HIV as sexual partners to be a discriminatory and ethically dubious practice. Despite this, he felt compelled to serosort because of fear.

'I found a big thing with me afterwards [after starting to use PrEP]. I'm not discriminating! I'm not! ... On the odd occasions when I did have bareback sex before, I would always ask. I don't want to ask someone their status, but I would turn around and say, 'I'm HIV-negative' when I last had a test, so-and-so, and encourage them to volunteer. Yeah, I was trying to serosort, which in a way – which is discriminating in a way. I found since going on PrEP, it doesn't matter and I'm not discriminating anymore. [I am] meeting people I wouldn't have been close to, friendly to, in the past.' (Allan)

Allan used to feel uncomfortable asking explicitly about a partner's HIV status, because he did not want to be seen as discriminating against people living with HIV. PrEP effectively removed the need for that conversation, and Allan believed this opened up the possibility to connect sexually with men living with HIV. Of course, the goal was not simply to have sex with men from a larger pool of possible partners, but rather to stop a practice that Allan felt was ethically problematic and excluded HIV-positive men. When seen in the larger context of Allan's earlier activism and the community AIDS trauma, it becomes evident that the possibility to comfortably discontinue serosorting had profound significance.

Notably, the construction of a serodivide, understood as a barrier separating people living with HIV from those who are HIV-negative, does not have to be a deliberate or malicious practice for its community-dividing effects to become destructive. Allan acknowledged this divide, and observed that PrEP finally afforded him the confidence to discontinue serosorting. There is research supporting the notion that PrEP may facilitate bridging the serodivide (Koester et al, 2018), a fact appreciated by the communities of people living with HIV (NAPWHA, 2019). In fact, PrEP may allow an

HIV 'status neutral' partner selection, and Canadian data (Wang et al, 2019) suggests that gay PrEP users select partners from pools of HIV-positive and HIV-negative men at rates approximately proportionate to their numbers in the community; such patterns contrast with the practices of PrEP non-users, who often serosort.

From Allan's perspective, PrEP's role in bridging the serodivide achieved much more than simply expanding the pool of possible sexual partners. It mended the community that was broken by the AIDS crisis, helped to include men living with HIV among those who could belong on an intimate level, and enabled unfettered connection with men of any HIV status.

Conclusion

For Allan, the arrival of PrEP marked the beginning of a new era in gay men's sexual health and well-being: for the very first time the joy of the pre-AIDS sexual experience was combined with social advancements of gay rights. Allan clearly remembered the time when gay men did not use condoms at all, as these were reserved for preventing unwanted pregnancy. The AIDS epidemic, however, caused a substantial change in practices of the gay community and led Allan to start using condoms consistently. Of course, the need to use condoms and the meanings they entailed had an impact on Allan's relationships and the feelings of connectedness with other men. Physical intimacy with other men was contaminated by fear of transmission of a deadly virus, and feelings of doubt, mistrust and insecurity started to accompany his encounters.

The introduction of PrEP had a profound transformative effect on Allan's sexual well-being. He was able, once again, to experience the 'unlimited' (Dean, 2009) joy and pleasure from connecting with other men and experiencing greater intimacy. Discontinuing condom use enabled him to realise that sexual connectedness was a way for him to achieve meaningful social connection with other men. He noticed that PrEP gave him the confidence to stop serosorting his partners, a practice that he saw as exclusionary and difficult to justify from an ethical standpoint. The new perspective allowed Allan to discover how deeply his sexual experiences had been affected by the fear of HIV. Sex with other men used to be associated with feelings of guilt and shame, and these extended long beyond the given encounter. PrEP replaced these emotions with the feeling of pure pleasure and recovered an important function of sexual experience – transcending the boundaries of individuality in connection with a partner. Allan was happy that he was able to see these changes, and he felt he was able to fully appreciate them because of his rich life experience. Allan considered these effects of PrEP to be life-changing.

In the history of HIV prevention discourses, there has been a narrative of opposition between the relative acceptability and safety of sanitised sex with condoms and the terror of transgressing the established boundaries. At the same time, the inherently transgressive, defiant nature of same-sex desire was ignored, despite this being strongly implicated in the construction of gay identity (Crossley, 2002). With the privatisation and domestication of gay experience to better suit the assimilationist project (for example, gay marriage), problematic sexual practices were removed from sight and cast out to the margins of gay culture (see, for example, Weiss, 2008, on BDSM – bondage, discipline, sadism and masochism – communities). To earn the social acceptance of gay normality, the newly emerged mainstreamed gay culture used shame to abject and police the practices and agents who did not fit into the categories of rationality and social desirability (Duggan, 2002; Weiss, 2008; Hindman, 2019). The tension between these two contradictory aspects of the gay habitus (transgression versus homonormative assimilation) manifested with the ambivalence around condomless sex, which was both desired and despised.

In Allan's story, PrEP was instrumental in reconciling these opposing elements of the gay identity. While condomless sex was still, at a deeper level, seen as transgressive of the symbolic boundaries and a forbidden fruit, PrEP allowed it to also become a reasonable, and safer, alternative to the imperative of consistent condom use. It removed the symbolic boundary established by condoms and enabled Allan to have his sexual desire actualised completely.

Allan's story shows that older gay men may greatly benefit from novel methods of prevention, not only from the HIV prevention standpoint but also in terms of increased sexual satisfaction. Inclusion of men belonging to the AIDS generation in all aspects of modern combination prevention that includes PrEP provision and promotion (United Nations General Assembly, 2021) may provide significant benefits to their quality of life and restore satisfying and meaningful sexual connections in a safe fashion. This may have consequences for counselling and care for older gay men, whose sexual satisfaction should be considered as one of the axes of well-being. Access to novel methods of HIV prevention should be assured on a level comparable to that of younger men, including in residential care, to ensure sexual autonomy and well-being as important components of sexual health.

References

Altman, D. (2013) *The End of the Homosexual?* Saint Lucia, Australia: University of Queensland Press.

Aspin, C. (2007) 'Takatāpui – confronting demonisation', in J. Hutchings and C. Aspin (eds) *Sexuality & the Stories of Indigenous People*, Wellington, New Zealand: Huia, pp 159–67.

Batza, K. (2018) *Before AIDS: Gay Health Politics in the 1970s*, Philadelphia, PA: University of Pennsylvania Press.

Bawer, B. (1993) *A Place at the Table: The Gay Individual in American Society*, New York: Poseidon Press.

BBC (2021) 'Homosexuality: the countries where it is illegal to be gay' [online], Available from: https://www.bbc.com/news/world-43822234

Bennett, J. (2009) 'Keeping the Wolfenden from the door? Homosexuality and the "medical model" in New Zealand', *Social History of Medicine*, 23(1): 134–52.

Bourdieu, P. (1977) *Outline of a Theory of Practice*, Cambridge: Cambridge University Press.

Bower, K.L., Lewis, D.C., Bermúdez, J.M. and Singh, A.A. (2019) 'Narratives of generativity and resilience among LGBT older adults: leaving positive legacies despite social stigma and collective trauma', *Journal of Homosexuality*, 68(2): 1–22.

BPAC NZ (2019) 'HIV pre-exposure prophylaxis (PrEP): a how-to guide' [online], Available from: https://bpac.org.nz/2019/prep.aspx

Brashers, D.E., Neidig, J.L., Cardillo, L.W., Dobbs, L.K., Russell, J.A. and Haas, S.M. (1999) '"In an important way, I did die": uncertainty and revival in persons living with HIV or AIDS', *AIDS Care*, 11(2): 201–19.

Brinkmann, S. (2014) 'Doing without data', *Qualitative Inquiry*, 20(6): 720–5.

Crossley, M.L. (2002) 'The perils of health promotion and the "barebacking" backlash', *Health*, 6(1): 47–68.

Crossley, M.L. (2004) 'Making sense of "barebacking": gay men's narratives, unsafe sex and the "resistance habitus"', *British Journal of Social Psychology*, 43(2): 225–44.

Crossley, M.L. (2007) 'Response to commentaries for "Making sense of 'barebacking': gay men's narratives, unsafe sex and 'resistance habitus'"', *British Journal of Social Psychology*, 46(3): 691–5.

Davis, P. (ed) (1996) *Intimate Details and Vital Statistics: AIDS, Sexuality and the Social Order in New Zealand*, Auckland, New Zealand: Auckland University Press.

Dean, T. (2009) *Unlimited Intimacy: Reflections on the Subculture of Barebacking*, Chicago, IL: University of Chicago Press.

Debesay, J., Nåden, D. and Slettebø, Å. (2008) 'How do we close the hermeneutic circle? A Gadamerian approach to justification in interpretation in qualitative studies', *Nursing Inquiry*, 15(1): 57–66.

Dickson, N., Lee, B., Foster, T. and Saxton, P.J. (2015) 'The first 30 years of HIV in New Zealand: review of the epidemiology', *New Zealand Medical Journal*, 128(1426): 31–48.

Duggan, L. (2002) 'The new homonormativity: the sexual politics of neoliberalism', in R. Castronovo and D.D. Nelson (eds) *Materializing Democracy: Toward a Revitalized Cultural Politics*, Durham, NC: Duke University Press, pp 175–94.

Elder, G.H., Johnson, M.K. and Crosnoe, R. (2003) 'The emergence and development of life course theory', in J.T. Mortimer and M.J. Shanahan (eds) *Handbook of the Life Course*, Boston, MA: Springer, pp 3–19.

Gadamer, H.-G. (1975) *Truth and Method*, London: Sheed & Ward.

Garcia, C. (2013) 'Limited intimacy: barebacking and the imaginary', *Textual Practice*, 27(6): 1031–51.

Gardiner, B. (2018) 'Grit and stigma: gay men ageing with HIV in regional Queensland', *Journal of Sociology*, 54(2): 214–25.

Grierson, J. and Smith, A.M.A. (2005) 'In from the outer: generational differences in coming out and gay identity formation', *Journal of Homosexuality*, 50(1): 53–70.

Grierson, J., Pitts, M., Herewini, T.H., Rua'ine, G., Hughes, A. J., Saxton, P.J.W., Whyte, M., Misson, S. and Thomas, M. (2004) 'Mate aaraikore a muri ake nei: experiences of Māori New Zealanders living with HIV', *Sexual Health*, 1(3): 175–80.

Halkitis, P.N. (2014) *The AIDS Generation: Stories of Survival and Resilience*, Oxford: Oxford University Press.

Halkitis, P.N. (2019) *Out in Time: The Public Lives of Gay Men from Stonewall to the Queer Generation*, New York: Oxford University Press.

Hammack, P.L., Frost, D.M., Meyer, I.H. and Pletta, D.R. (2018) 'Gay men's health and identity: social change and the life course', *Archives of Sexual Behavior*, 47(1): 59–74.

Hammack, P.L., Toolis, E.E., Wilson, B.D.M., Clark, R.C. and Frost, D.M. (2019) 'Making meaning of the impact of pre-exposure prophylaxis (PrEP) on public health and sexual culture: narratives of three generations of gay and bisexual men', *Archives of Sexual Behaviour*, 48, 1041–58.

Henrickson, M. (2006) 'Kō wai ratou? Managing multiple identities in lesbian, gay and bisexual New Zealand Māori', *New Zealand Sociology*, 21(2): 247–69.

Hindman, M.D. (2019) 'Promiscuity of the past: neoliberalism and gay sexuality pre- and post-AIDS', *Politics, Groups, and Identities*, 7(1): 52–70.

Holmes, D. and Warner, D. (2005) 'The anatomy of a forbidden desire: men, penetration and semen exchange', *Nursing Inquiry*, 12(1): 10–20.

Kirby, M. (2008) 'Lessons from the Wolfenden Report', *Commonwealth Law Bulletin*, 34(3): 551–9.

Koester, K.A., Erguera, X.A., Kang Dufour, M.-S., Udoh, I., Burack, J.H., Grant, R.M. and Myers, J.J. (2018) '"Losing the phobia": understanding how HIV pre-exposure prophylaxis facilitates bridging the serodivide among men who have sex with men', *Frontiers in Public Health* [online], 6: 250. doi: 10.3389/fpubh.2018.00250

Laverty, S.M. (2003) 'Hermeneutic phenomenology and phenomenology: a comparison of historical and methodological considerations', *International Journal of Qualitative Methods*, 2(3): 21–35.

Lindberg, W. and McMorland, J. (1996) '"From grassroots to business suits": the gay community response to AIDS', in P. Davis (ed) *Intimate Details and Vital Statistics: AIDS, Sexuality and the Social Order in New Zealand*, Auckland, New Zealand: Auckland University Press, pp 102–20.

NAPWHA (National Association of People with HIV Australia) (2019) 'What does PrEP mean for people with HIV?' [online], Available from: https://napwha.org.au/wp-content/uploads/2019/02/NAPWHA-HIV-Pre-Exposure-Prophylaxis-PrEP.pdf

Palella, F.J., Delaney, K.M., Moorman, A.C., Loveless, M.O., Fuhrer, J., Satten, G.A., Aschman, D.J. and Holmberg, S.D. (1998) 'Declining morbidity and mortality among patients with advanced human immunodeficiency virus infection', *New England Journal of Medicine*, 338: 853–60.

Parkinson, P. and Hughes, T. (1987) 'The gay community and the response to AIDS in New Zealand', *New Zealand Medical Journal*, 100: 77–9.

Paul, R. (2012) 'Hans-Georg Gadamer's philosophical hermeneutics: concepts of reading, understanding and interpretation', *Meta: Research in Hermeneutics, Phenomenology and Practical Philosophy*, 4(2): 286–303.

Prevention Access Campaign (2016) 'Risk of sexual transmission of HIV from a person living with HIV who has undetectable viral load. Messaging primer & consensus statement' [online], Available from: https://www.preventionaccess.org/consensus

Rofes, E. (1998) *Dry Bones Breathe: Gay Men Creating Post-AIDS Identities and Cultures*, New York: Routledge.

Rua'ine, G. (2007) 'Takatāpui and HIV – a personal journey', in J. Hutchings and C. Aspin (eds) *Sexuality and the Stories of Indigenous People*, Wellington, New Zealand: Huia, pp 149–58.

Shilts, R. (1988) *And the Band Played On: Politics, People, and the AIDS Epidemic*, New York: Penguin Books.

United Nations General Assembly (2021) *Political Declaration on HIV and AIDS: Ending Inequalities and Getting on Track to End AIDS by 2030*, Geneva: UNAIDS, Available from: https://www.unaids.org/en/resources/documents/2021/2021_political-declaration-on-hiv-and-aids

Wang, L., Moqueet, N., Lambert, G., Grace, D., Rodrigues, R., Cox, J., Lachowsky, N.J., Noor, S.W., Armstrong, H.L., Tan, D.H.S., Burchell, A.N., Ma, H., Apelian, H., Knight, J., Messier-Peet, M., Jollimore, J., Baral, S., Hart, T.A., Moore, D.M. and Mishra, S. (2019) 'Population-level sexual mixing by HIV status and pre-exposure prophylaxis use among men who have sex with men in Montréal, Canada: implications for HIV prevention', *American Journal of Epidemiology*, 189(1): 44–54.

Weiss, M.D. (2008) 'Gay shame and BDSM pride: neoliberalism, privacy, and sexual politics', *Radical History Review*, 2008(100): 86–101.

Wells, N. (2020) 'PrEP, risk and sexual behaviours: PrEP users' critiques of "risk compensation" language', *Joint Australasian HIV&AIDS and Sexual Health Conferences*, Virtual, 16–20 November 2020, Available from: https://az659834.vo.msecnd.net/eventsairaueprod/production-ashm-public/0402bb6c703a426895245426afeb23db

6

In the company of men: gay culture and HIV in Aotearoa New Zealand

Michael Stevens

Memory is an unreliable guide, so they say, and as Joni Mitchell (1975) put it: 'Every picture has its shadows, and it has some source of light.' I write as a White HIV-positive gay cisgender man, born and living in Aotearoa New Zealand, approaching my sixties. New Zealand is geographically part of the Global South and today much more aware of its Indigenous culture and our place in the Pacific than in my youth, but economically and culturally more aligned to the Global North, to Europe and North America rather than to Africa, Asia or South America. This fact also shapes my experiences.

In my late teens, I lived in Australia; in my twenties, I spent eight months in the United States and then eight years in Turkey. AIDS nearly killed me a couple of times. I am aware of my privilege, and I frame my writing here with that background. I do not pretend to tell a universal story, but believe there are aspects of my own story that will resonate with others. I hope what I am exploring here will add to our understanding of how we as gay men got to where we are now, from the pre-AIDS days and through the worst of that catastrophe to the world we are in today. I want to write about sex, about HIV, about culture and ageing within it.

There used to be a Pride centre here in Auckland, that had a library, a big library. It was largely made up of books from men who had died of AIDS.

There were multiple copies of some books, and I still have some of these on my own shelves.

The Front Runner. Faggots. Dancer from the Dance. Maurice. Lovers: The Story of Two Men. Giovanni's Room. Our Lady of the Flowers, to name a few.

One younger gay man I know recently said *Faggots* blew his mind. He'd never realised such a world existed. He found it and loved it.

One reason there were multiple copies is that in New Zealand in the 1970s these books were so hard to get, and one place you could get them was the Out! bookshop, attached to the office of the magazine of the same name. They had a captive market, thus many of us bought and read the same books, and kept them. If they trusted you, they'd even let you buy porn they somehow smuggled in.

They always had a sandwich board outside with that month's cover model on it, usually a typical semi-clothed beefcake in the woods or on a beach, with the strapline 'the alternative lifestyle'. For months I walked past and ogled those men, thinking 'alternative lifestyle' must be something to do with hiking and mountaineering. I'm not sure how I finally figured it out, to be honest.

Even going into this space, up a narrow staircase on a side street, to a dingy little office, took courage. What if someone saw you? How would you explain it?

They had an odd assortment of books, from things like *Giovanni's Room*, which you could probably have bought in a big bookshop, to more niche but popular works like *The Front Runner* to collections of poetry (I bought Felice Picano's *The Deformity Lover and Other Poems* there in 1979) and plays and anthologies translated from Spanish. I also bought a first edition of *The Joy of Gay Sex*, which I wish I still had. They cast a wide net, because they were trying to get anything and everything gay that they could. And because we were so starved of anything, we bought what was there.

The hunger to have something, anything, that told our stories, that reflected us back, was huge. It's so hard to explain today, and I know how people complain about the lack of representation on TV and in movies and popular culture, but back then it was a desert!

To be so invisible, yet to know we existed, to know I existed, was such a contradiction, traumatic in many ways. So finding anything that validated, that represented, that spoke to my gayness, to my otherness, to my wholeness, was essential.

I think it was so for many other gay men too, and that's why I recognised so many of those dead men's books. Books that had been important to them, as they had been to me, books that had offered a mirror, or a view of possibilities, of other lives.

This odd collection of books was one of the ways I learned to be a gay man.

No wonder so many gay men from New Zealand had a history of leaving this country in our twenties. We wanted to breathe. We wanted to be in cities that had gay ghettoes. We wanted to live in a world that we had only been able to read about.

Another way I learned to be gay was through my body, through lust, desire, and through love.

I became sexually active with other men at around the age of 15 – I can't quite recall the exact age – and told my parents I was gay when I was 17. I went to university at 18 and became involved with Gay Liberation on campus. I had always known I was 'different', but it was puberty that showed me just what that meant. Back in the 1970s, being gay in New Zealand was illegal, and also scorned in a way that is hard to describe today.

I often say I grew up in saunas and public toilets.

My first sexual experience with a man was in a public toilet. No planning on my part, I went in for a pee and saw this man masturbating there. I left and went about what I was doing, then came back and he was still there, and we went into a cubicle and had sex. I wanted to. I already knew I was gay. I knew what men's bodies meant to me. I wasn't raped, I wanted sex, though today I shake my head in bemusement at my 15(or so)-year-old self being so brave and foolish.

And once I was 16, I started going to the local sauna, or a bathhouse in American. They actually had an age restriction – probably sensible, but seeing everything that went on there was illegal at the time, it seems a bit pointless in retrospect.

The fact we had to have these separate, clandestine places to meet says much in itself. We emphasised the 'sex' in homosexual.

I was having lots and lots of sex. It seems, looking back, that we all were. In public toilets, in saunas, picking up in clubs and bars, in parks, cruising on the street. Sex, it seemed, was the main point of being gay.

The third way I learned to be gay was through activism, through finding my community and my people. I went on my first Gay Liberation protest in 1979, during my first year at university. I met people who challenged my ideas of the status quo, who talked of different ways we could be. I read Marx. I read feminist writers. I read more and more gay writers. And I had sex with some of these activist friends – these threads in my life of sex, literature and activism entwined to form something stronger. This added a layer of interpretation and understanding to my experiences as well as connecting me with a wider set of gay men and, for the first time, lesbians. Some of them are still friends to this day. So the social and political came to weave through physical lust and literature.

I tease and trace these threads of how I learned to become gay, because these experiences shaped me and relate directly to how I became HIV-positive. And I believe that my story has commonalities with many of my contemporaries. We had to learn how to become gay. We succeeded. Then just as everything seemed wonderful and on the verge of a new dawn, we had to learn something else.

Why did the books matter so much, and what could I, a teenager in New Zealand, learn from them, set, as they mostly were, in the United States or the United Kingdom, and some, like *Maurice*, from a time before I was born, others from before I came out? I have been rereading them now as I write this, some for the first time in decades, and they still speak to me, because they speak of great themes, especially the quest for love, and the way we gay men tend to conflate lust for love, or to take the easy availability of sexual intimacy over the more difficult work of emotional intimacy. Yet under all that fucking, so clearly, so often, most of us really wanted love.

These books mattered because they showed possibilities that could lead to love, to joy, to pride. Winston Leyland, the pioneering editor of the Gay Sunshine Press anthology *Orgasms of Light*, coined the term 'Gay Cultural Renaissance' and wrote:

> When literary historians look back on this period of letters in a hundred years from now I firmly believe they will view this Gay Cultural Renaissance as being of equal importance to other literary movements (such as the Beat) of the second half of the 20th century. (Leyland, 1977, p 9)

I am not sure he was right, but his vision in 1977 was one of immense optimism and possibility, and belief in the power of social change through literature. In my personal life, and I think the wider cultural zeitgeist for gay men, these books mattered.

Sex mattered because it had been forbidden for so long. The simple act of two men making love, or just having some fun, was illegal in my own country until I was 25, and longer in other similar countries. It is an act that can still result in imprisonment, torture and death in a number of countries today.

Sex matters because it is fun, and when done well, more than fun – it takes us to a place of physical ecstasy, and many gay men prided and still pride themselves on being sexual athletes in a positive sense.

Sex matters because the act of men delighting in sodomy is a direct affront to the patriarchal notion of what it is to be a man.

Sex matters because for so long, and even today to a large extent, the difference of our sex acts is what is used by the mainstream to define us.

Two men fucking is a political act. Still.

I still remember a long hot and steamy night in a sauna in Melbourne, in a mirrored room. I was 19, and he was in his early twenties and in the army. We were there for hours, together, in every way possible. Joyous, joyful, taking breaks and talking between sex. I never saw him again, but I remember him with real affection.

Like many gay men, I made a distinction between fucking for fun and making love. Sometimes the edges blur between these, but for many of us, sex for fun was an activity as normal as playing a game of tennis. A recreation, something that had no strings, no consequences. Sometimes played with friends, more often played with strangers. And something that felt subversive of the norm, rule-breaking.

Sex matters because it is one of the deepest ways to reveal ourselves to those we love. At its best, it is a time of vulnerability, of openness, of exposing ourselves to another.

Holleran's *Dancer from the Dance* is a book I fell in love with. It showed me a world, and it was a real world, a culture. It infatuated me, and I looked for it and found bits of it in New York, in London, even traces of it here in New Zealand. It represented glamour, decadence, sex and, most of all, love. As well as the decadence, though, there was a self-awareness to it. One of the final letters between the men telling the story of Malone observes how when their group of night-clubbing, drug-taking, sex-driven friends took part in a New York gay liberation march, they were stunned to see all the men they didn't know, to realise that there was an entire world of gay, lesbian and queer people out there who weren't part of 'the scene'. That's a tension that still exists today.

This book, and Kramer's *Faggots*, along with Edmund White's *A Boy's Own Story* a little bit later, all showed this young uncertain gay man from New Zealand a world that was out there waiting to be found, a world I could relate to, and that shaped me in some ways. These books were fiction but closely built on reality. And they emphasised sex in such a way – the joy of it, the freedom of it, the sadness and futility that can come with it too.

To reread them now is to look at a world that has gone, but one for which I feel enormous affection. This was the world I was supposed to move into. A world of gay men, to a large extent, where we centred our lives on nonconformity, on joy and satisfaction. This makes sense to me because so much else that was publicly associated with being gay was so negative, so scared and sad. These stories were so defiant, so poignant, so tender, so real and, with all the faults of their worlds, so true.

These books portrayed an emerging urban gay culture. A world of men that was free, fun and proud. They nearly all came from the United States, so it might seem odd they had so much power, but America has defined popular culture for so long and this is what made them so powerful. To hear these voices and stories coming from the country that gave us Disney, MGM (Metro-Goldwyn-Mayer), so much of our TV – this gave them authenticity. They showed possibilities that sleepy provincial New Zealand could not offer.

Sex was central. So many of these writers, and so many of the activists who created this world for us through gay liberation, were baby boomers, and in the 1970s and 1980s when these books came out, they were in their twenties and thirties. They were young men experiencing the thrill of being able to live a new kind of life, and I wanted that too.

I still remember going home with one man, probably in his forties. He'd picked me up in a public toilet in town in the middle of the day, and we went back to his house. I could tell immediately it was a family home, and when we got to the bedroom, he turned a wedding photo face down before we got to it.

When I look back now, I took incredible risks, but they didn't seem risky to me, because I didn't realise just how bad the world could be.

So my young gay self was shaped by sex. And books. And by activism.

Before my first year at university started, I went over a few times, ostensibly to familiarise myself with the place but really to look out for any signals of gay life. I checked the catalogue in the library and found 'Homosexuality', which I think was 301.4-something in the Dewey system. I took a lift to the appropriate floor and hunted the position out. It was meagre, maybe one shelf, about two or three feet long, of books. But to me it was a cornucopia. The title I remember most clearly is Katz's *Gay American History* – I was just blown away that anyone would write gay history! Of a country! And I was holding the book in my hands in a library! How do I explain how revolutionary this was? Again, it was a sign of being seen, being recognised, being valid.

On one of those visits to that bookshelf, I looked down the library aisle and there was a tall, handsome young guy standing there. I looked at the books I was examining then took a second glance. He had his cock out and was jerking off looking at me. We went to the men's room and had sex. Books and sex! Books as a way to get sex! My two favourite things!

I could go on with many similar anecdotes, but what strikes me is the way gay sex was illegal, yet it was there, so ready to be found, if you knew how to look or stumbled across the right places. And it was different from hooking up today on an app. You had to be less picky for one thing, and you were exposed to a very wide range of men of all types and ages.

So for me, my late teens and early twenties were full of fucking, and I loved it. I also longed for a boyfriend, or thought I did. I remember one of the guys in a couple I had sex with a few times telling me I didn't need a boyfriend yet, just a fuck buddy. That was the first time I'd heard that term. I ended up with a few. Many friends were made and a few lost through all this fun.

I was already gay, I already lusted after men and had done with the awakening of my sexual feelings – but I learned how to be gay through a mix of praxis and literature, fictional and academic.

This shaped me in so many ways, ways I still examine and look to understand.

I had a community based in those three imaginings and activities. Activism, sex, and literature all linked to and fed each other.

My story is not that unusual though. I know this. Many of my contemporaries undertook similar voyages of discovery and reward. I am a little unusual in still being here.

In the gay world that I knew before HIV/AIDS, the 'scene' was orgiastic, free and intensely liberating from the fear, shame and uncertainty I'd felt before. I remember being told at around the age of 18 that one of the great things about being gay was we could have much sex as we liked and nothing bad would happen. No unwanted babies, no expectations that sex meant marriage. And free sex was seen as liberating, a political act, something that challenged the patriarchy and ideas of how men should behave. Being in an orgy of similar aged youth was as innocent and as fun as a pile of puppies crawling over each other and playing.

I look at my younger self and am glad of the experiences I had. I'm proud of them. There seems such innocence to it all.

We weren't afraid of our bodies. We weren't afraid of sex. We weren't afraid of each other. We didn't potentially carry disease and death within us, that we could pass on. How that changed.

I have some journals from those days from before the plague, and looking back at the young me, I feel distance, and compassion.

Along with everything else in my life, I longed for love. So many entries about hoping this man will love me, or that one. That I will find happiness. While it is somewhat painful to look back at these memories, entries I haven't looked at in decades, the almost universal desire to love and be loved is real, and that too ties into all that happened before, during and after the plague.

Before HIV, sex was innocent, largely celebratory, and had no threat of illness and death.

After HIV, that innocence was lost. And death and sex were mingled together in a way that was a direct affront on the world we had created and the one I grew up in.

How could something so sweet, so fun, so central to our being become suddenly so deadly? It was as if all the stories that religious zealots and other homophobes had threatened us with for years suddenly materialised.

I remember in San Francisco, in 1984, staying at an apartment of Radical Faeries in the Haight. One of the guys there sat me down and got me very stoned and told me about all the men he knew who had got sick and died in the last few years. One of his friends had dressed himself up in his full BDSM (bondage, discipline, sadism and masochism) leather regalia and gone and hanged himself from a tree in his neighbourhood park when he realised he was getting sick. The storyteller was trying to scare me safe.

It was so hard to understand at first. I met a man in New York, another New Zealander, in 1985 who said he hadn't had sex for two years. He was too terrified. I didn't really understand. The gay scene was still going when I was there, but it was slowly collapsing, though I didn't know it. Back here in New Zealand, there were rumours of friends getting sick, dying. We had no internet then and international phone calls were a luxury. So rumours came, whispers of what was happening.

But part of why I was travelling in the US and the world was to take part in that banquet of flesh, to be both fed and food, to live out at least in part some of the stories I'd read. And I did.

In 1984 I fucked my way from San Francisco to New York, then spent another seven months or so living and working illegally there. With hindsight, not the best time to be doing what I was doing. The New St Marks Baths were still open, as was the Mineshaft, the Saint and the Anvil, though they all closed not long after I left in 1985.

I moved on to live in Turkey for eight years. It is hard to capture how isolating that felt. With no internet, no mobile phones, no instant communications across the globe, we relied on letters and the occasional expensive phone call to stay in contact. Rumours of more friends' deaths came through.

But, I seemed to be fine. And I was. But then my flatmate, an English guy working in the same school as me, didn't come home for a couple of nights, and we eventually traced him to a hospital. He had tuberculosis. Shortly after he was well enough to come home, he flew back to London for an HIV test. He was positive. This was 1988. And this made me face up for the first time to the possibility that I might be as well. So in my summer break I took off to London for a test as well. I went to a free clinic but because I had no UK citizenship rights, I couldn't get a test. A doctor listened to my story and told me I probably had it, and had about two years left to live. I was 27.

I ended up going to a private clinic to get tested, which confirmed my fears. And it felt like my world had ended.

I decided to stay on in Turkey. I did this as I wasn't actually sick, and I made sure I had enough money to get back to New Zealand in a hurry if I had to.

In 1992 one of my best friends came to visit. He'd been one of the first people I knew to be diagnosed with HIV. He was very sick and making a farewell tour of friends before he died. When he did die a few months later, it made me think it was time to return, so I did.

The gay world I'd left had changed immeasurably. We were now legal, for one thing. No more being outlaws. And the men I knew who were still alive were fighting for their lives, and the lives of their friends and lovers. The great gay cultural renaissance seemed to be coming down in flames around us.

Sex became fraught, dangerous, filled with the potential that ecstasy could bring death. And it did for so many. One friend still has his 'funeral suit' even though it doesn't fit now. He can't part with it – he wore it to so many.

I got sick, very sick. I couldn't walk at one stage because I couldn't breathe enough. Sex disappeared out of my life. I was angry. How could my body, this source of untold delight and pleasure, turn against me? How did any of this make sense?

So the thread of sex in my life weakened.

But the other two threads, of literature and activism, remained. There was now a new literary rush, of AIDS memoirs and fiction, and I devoured them hungrily. I wonder now what they would be like to revisit.

And activism again gave me community. Fighting for access to medications, organising, running support groups and getting politically engaged. I went from going to an HIV peer-support group to becoming a facilitator for several and being on the board of Body Positive, an organisation run by and for people living with HIV/AIDS. We never had an ACT UP here, but we did have a Treatment Action Group for a while, and I was the last director of that before it shut. Later I became chair of the New Zealand AIDS Foundation, a role that moved my activism into the mainstream.

The growing body of AIDS literature reinforced the role of literature in forming myself. A lot of these works were from overseas, such as Feinberg's *Eighty-Sixed*, White's *The Farewell Symphony* or Hollinghurst's *The Line of Beauty*, but local works, such as the late Douglas Wright's memoir *Ghost Dance*, had a strong impact.

And if I too had often substituted sex for love, where now would I find love? That seems impossible. Who would or could love someone who carried this virus? It was a bleak and lonely time of my life in that regard, though filled with friendship and other good things. But love, the dream I'd had since young, to love and be loved by a good man – this now seemed impossible, and I was resigned to dying alone.

HIV/AIDS had such a shattering effect on the world we thought we were creating. The social and communal worlds of gay men were radically upended. It was like standing in the ruins after a bomb blast or an earthquake and trying to figure out what had happened. So many things we treasured were destroyed; so many that we loved, dead.

And when I say three threads taught me how to be gay – literature, sex and activism – there is the fourth one. AIDS. It didn't teach me how to be gay, but since my diagnosis it has shaped so much of my life, taught me so much, even when it removed so much of my precious autonomy, taught me that I can't have everything, that life is hard and ugly, as well as beautiful.

Now, nearly 60, I live and work and I love and am loved. I am lucky. But the world of young queers seems so different to mine in so many ways. Perhaps this is the normal generational difference that occurs. But their world wasn't shaped in the way mine was. We often seem to talk past each other rather than to each other. The world that I think we thought we were creating back in my youth was derailed and destroyed.

Yet I am still a gay man, and when I talk with younger gay men, I find myself wondering "Is being gay in itself enough to create an understanding in the way it used to be?" When we had no positive visibility, when we were illegal, we had to get along and support each other somehow. That seems to have gone, or perhaps I am simply not connected to it any longer in the ways I once was. In the world of today's queer activists, it seems age is not welcome. Just as we become invisible on the scene when we get too old, just as all the beautiful muscle boys and bright young things ignore us, so too do the activists of today it seems. Our concerns are irrelevant, and we should move out of the way. So it often seems.

This disconnect between the pain we went through and the way this time has been lost to the collective memory of our youth still surprises me.

But then, we did lose a large part of a generation of people. Of artists and writers, activists and leaders, and ordinary men who wanted to live and to love. They are not here to pass down all that knowledge.

My body is ageing. After all the physical horrors AIDS inflicted on me, now I find the indignities of old age are creeping up instead. This is not something I was expecting. And as I didn't expect to live, I didn't plan for any future, so now it seems my old age will be financially difficult.

What does sex mean to me now? It is something I think about much more than I do. Being loved, in a relationship, I delight in the shared intimacy of physical contact beyond sex.

It becomes hard to disentangle the facts that now govern my sex life. Is it age? Is it the fact that many HIV-positive men have lowered testosterone? I don't know how to separate these things. Have I grown to see sex as a less defining part of who I am? I think that is part of it.

I have long believed the thing that really makes us gay is our desire to fully love and be loved by the same sex, not just the sex acts themselves. Now that I have that love and intimacy in my life, sex has receded in importance. Or, I ask myself, is it age? Or the effects of HIV?

Up until this relationship, I was still very sexually active. I had my regular fuck buddies. I explored the limits of kink and BDSM, a theme that had always been present in my sex life. I was busy on the apps.

Earlier, after diagnosis, sex had become forbidden and forbidding. Instead of the joyful free-for-all, it was now freighted with sickness, shame and death. Safe sex was a great idea and could be good, but stopping to put on a condom always robbed the moment of something. To disclose or not to disclose? Even when having strictly safe sex, this sat there as a huge obstacle. (Note: in New Zealand there is no legal obligation to disclose, only to take all reasonable precautions to protect.)

So as the data came in to show having an undetectable viral load meant we were unable to pass the virus on, this was welcomed with great pleasure. I resumed fucking as I felt like it. I was much older and physically not as desirable to most men as I had been in my youth, but I could still get laid, still have fun. And I did.

My body was once a source of pure physical joy and delight. I had a sense of sexual prowess and athleticism. I was proud of how good I was at sex. I put in a lot of practice.

Then my body became something I could not trust, something that could harm and kill others. Guilt and fear destroyed so much that had once been simply fun.

Now it is something again that is not what it was, something that still always carries a shadow, but can, if I wish it, return to something close to the freedom and ecstasy I so enjoyed in my youth.

But there is no doubt that AIDS has changed what sex means to me, and it will never be the same. I miss that. I miss the uninhibited carnivalesque joy of my sexual youth. Even while rationally knowing that I cannot infect others, there is still a voice in my head that goes, "but what if?"

Age is a factor. Western society focuses desire on the young. Middle-aged heterosexual women talk of becoming invisible to men. It is the same for gay men, I believe. We do not fit the model that is marketed, we are not as desirable to most other same-sex attracted men. No number of campaign posters of physically desirable hot men who are out about living with the virus ever really reduces the stigma that is out there.

Age entwines with my HIV status as another factor that has changed what sex is to me. I cannot disentangle these elements, as much as I try at times, including while writing this.

The other question I ask myself is would my sex life now be different if I were HIV-negative and still this age, with this middle-aged body? I suspect not. In the harshly competitive way of modern gay culture, I am not the sex object I once enjoyed being.

But I am loved and I love. Deeply. I am engaged to a man who makes me laugh every day and who gives me so much strength and support. We met by chance, but clicked almost immediately. To be engaged and planning a wedding is something that seemed unimaginable in my youth. Indeed I remember going to a family wedding in my teens and crying at the thought that I would never have this sort of celebration of my love, that it was impossible. Now my family can't wait for us to actually tie the knot. My fiancé is positive too, which would have been more important 20 years ago than it is now, when the fear of infecting someone was so strong. Today it feels an incidental part of our relationship and who we are together.

As I wrote earlier, and I believe I am right, I think that the essence of being gay is not sex acts but our desire to love and be loved by those of the same sex. I am lucky to be in this place in my life now. Sex is not what binds us, though it is part of our relationship, but less so than if we were both younger. So as sex has receded in importance and centrality to my sense of self as a gay man, the ability to love openly has increased, and this gives me so much joy.

One of the unanswerable but important questions is, if we hadn't lost so much of that generation to AIDS, if we had all those millions of gay men around who had died, and if they had aged as I have, would we have created the world we dreamed of? Would Leyland's 'Gay Cultural Renaissance' have embedded itself into wider culture and created a world where gay men treat ageing differently?

Numbers matter: if there were that many more of us, the numbers that should have been, I do believe we would have much stronger and deeper communities. I also think that the loss of those men robbed us of much intergenerational richness, wisdom and continuity.

My life's trajectory surprises me, from the joy and exuberance of my youth, believing we were creating something vibrant, liberating and new, to the screaming pain and desperate exhaustion of the plague years, when we were just trying to stay alive, to now, when I am in many ways an ordinary ageing gay White man.

If, as it seemed in my youth, sex in itself was the main point of being gay, what does it mean to my life now that it is no longer so central? I go back to my contention that it is, and always was, love.

Yet the things that taught me to be gay – literature, sex and activism – continue in my life and continue to feed me. Even my HIV diagnosis does. These threads continue to weave core parts of my life. The one great desire I had as a young man, to truly, intimately love and be loved, is realised and continues to delight me in ways I never knew possible.

Writing this has been a challenge, forcing me to consider much. Some things are clear, some much less so. My story is personal, an autoethnographic look at what shaped me and brought me here. It is mine, but I believe it contains much that is recognisable to others of my generation – to other gay men who lived through what I have – and which I hope resonates with those younger gay men of today as well.

We had something special, we nearly lost it all, we found something else that was special. We continue.

Postscript: The collection of books I talked of at the start of this chapter was broken up and disposed of as "not our core business" by their last custodians. Our memory and culture, tenuous already, slowly dissipates through such actions driven by neoliberal logic.

References

Leyland, W. (1977) *Orgasms of Light*, San Francisco: Gay Sunshine Press.

Mitchell, J. (1975) *The Hissing of Summer Lawns* [CD], Los Angeles: A&M Records.

7

Growing old with stigma: a case study of four older Chinese gay/bisexual men living with HIV in Hong Kong

Barry Man Wai Lee 李文偉

Introduction

This chapter presents a qualitative study exploring the lived experiences of four older (over 60 years of age) Chinese gay/bisexual men living with HIV and how those experiences manifest in their lives in the Hong Kong context. Stories of the informants are explored during two periods of their lives. The first period (1950s to 1970s) concerns the time of their emerging sexuality; when most of their peers were engaged in heterosexual relationships, they attempted to remain unmarried while facing considerable pressure both from their families and society to conform. The second period (1990s to present day) relates to their diagnosis and living long-term with HIV. Their experiences of being non-heterosexual and living with HIV have been stigmatised because of cultural values related to their sexuality (for example, Confucian filial piety, familial obligation and loss of face) and shame about their illness.

In this study, informants' narratives are captured by means of face-to-face in-depth interviews. Four overarching themes emerged from the three areas of sexuality, HIV and ageing. First, the theme of 'filiality' captures how the informants handle their same-sex desires: playing along with both family and societal expectations to marry while also secretly exploring their same-sex attractions. Second, 'heterosexist harassment' reflects their experiences of facing both their own denial about their non-heterosexuality and the subtle/ indirect harassment from others. Third, 'hidden lives' focuses on how the informants negotiate their gay/bisexual and HIV identities in the context of home and the gay community. The fourth theme, 'living with ageing', considers how the informants cope with their sexuality and HIV during the process of ageing.

The findings show how the informants experience heterosexism, HIV stigma and ageism, compounded by the unique challenges they face both within the gay community and at a societal level. The narratives of the four older Chinese gay/bisexual men with HIV illustrate how their untold stories can shed a light on the intersectional area of sexuality, HIV and ageing stigma in Hong Kong.

Literature review

The term 'stigma' is defined by Goffman (1963) as 'a deeply discrediting attribute that globally devalues an individual' (p 12). Individuals' social identities are affected by attributes that mark them as deviant from social norms and as being incapable of fulfilling the role requirements of social interactions. As a result, individuals with stigmatised identity (identities) are systematically disadvantaged by the place that they occupy within society. Reviewing the relevant literature, it was found that older gay/bisexual with HIV are prone to several forms of stigma in the areas of ageing, sexuality and HIV.

Older people are susceptible to the impact of ageism. Ageism refers to a negative attitude towards ageing, often with a belief that older people are less attractive, less sexual or less cognitively competent (Atchley and Barusch, 2004). Older gay/bisexual men are often situated within a gay culture obsessed with youthfulness: certain body types seem prevalent, and ageism within the gay community is not uncommon (Slevin and Linneman, 2010; Gewirtz-Meydan et al, 2018). Hong Kong is no exception (Suen, 2017). For instance, Kong (2019) reveals ageism against one of his interviewees (a 65-year-old Chinese gay men), who was rejected when he tried to visit a gay sauna in Hong Kong, the excuse being that the sauna was for members only.

Experiences of stigma among older gay/bisexual men can be conceptualised as heterosexism, which refers to the normative assumptions that all people are heterosexuals and heterosexual orientation is the only normal and ideal form of sexuality (Herek, 1996). A study of healthcare professionals serving older adults identified a general assumption that service users were all heterosexual (Heaphy et al, 2003). Heterosexism can be understood on two levels. First, psychological heterosexism directs personal prejudice and biased behaviours, including verbal harassment and physical aggression, towards sexual minorities (Herek, 1995). Similar to the term 'homophobia', which refers to an irrational fear of male homosexuality (Weinberg, 1972), heterosexism highlights anti-gay sentiments at a psychological level; it is unlike phobias that manifest at a physiological level (Shields and Harriman, 1984). Heterosexist harassment, derived from heterosexism, is conceptualised as 'insensitive verbal and symbolic (but non-assaultive) behaviours that convey animosity toward non-heterosexuality' (Silverschanz et al, 2008, p 180). Heterosexist harassment captures both personal experiences of harassment – such as name-calling, using terms like 'faggot' – and heterosexist environments – created through, for example, telling anti-gay jokes. Anti-gay sentiments arising from heterosexism are rooted in cultural ideologies (Herek, 1990), therefore psychological heterosexism is often an individual manifestation of systemic attitudes. Second, cultural heterosexism can be promoted at social and institutional levels (Herek, 1996). In many instances, systemic discrimination towards sexual minorities is found within a society, including among older LGBT (lesbian, gay, bisexual and transgender) people (Woody, 2014).

Heterosexism does not occur in a vacuum. It can be influenced by historical, cultural, religious and legal constructs. Same-sex eroticism has been well documented within Chinese history (Ruan, 1991; Liu, 2003), and intimacy and sexual relationships between men were historically tolerated as long as filial obligations were maintained (Hinsch, 1990). Filiality, which is strongly influenced by Confucian beliefs, is the virtue of respect for parents. Within many Chinese cultures, getting married is an expression of filial piety (Dong and Xu, 2016). A majority of Hong Kong people are of Chinese descent, many of them coming from mainland China during the 1940s and 1950s. Confucianism is one of the most influential beliefs in Hong Kong society. British colonialisation and rule for over a century resulted in a hybrid of Eastern and Western cultures (Lu, 2009) in Hong Kong. The British Offences Against the Person Act of 1861, which criminalised male homosexual acts, was part of Hong Kong law until 1991 (Chou, 2000). In addition, fundamentalist religious condemnation of homosexuality and the medicalisation of homosexuality fuelled anti-gay sentiments within Hong Kong (Ng and Ma, 2004). Therefore homosexuality was considered immoral, unnatural, pathological and illegal (Ho, 1995), and as a result many older Chinese gay/bisexual men have endured negative experiences throughout their lives (Kong, 2019).

HIV stigma refers to the marginalisation or devaluation of people living with HIV. Apart from HIV's transmittable nature, particularly through sexual contact, and there being no cure when it was first identified in 1981 (Heyward and Curran, 1988), it is especially associated with certain stigmatised groups (including gay/bisexual men; Quinn and Earnshaw, 2011), behaviours (including anal sex; Kutner et al, 2020) and relationships (including those involving multiple sexual partners; Balzarini et al, 2018). Even though HIV stigma is not exclusive to gay/bisexual men, it tends to be associated with pre-existing stigma, such as those against gay/bisexual men, who are widely considered within society as abnormal, deviant and unnatural. When gay/bisexual men disclose their sexual orientation in public spaces, many experience harassment and/or discrimination in both subtle and significant ways (Herek, 2009). HIV stigma within the gay community was also documented when HIV antibody testing became available in 1985 (Sheon and Crosby, 2004), and stigma and discrimination against HIV-positive gay/bisexual men has remained prevalent within the community

(Smit et al, 2012). At the same time, research shows ambivalent attitudes of gay/bisexual men towards people living with HIV (Flowers et al, 2000). Thus, stigma management, such as concealment of stigmatised identity (Quinn and Earnshaw, 2011) or selective disclosure (Leask et al, 1997), are crucial survival skills for HIV-positive gay/bisexual men. Care and support are essential for all people living with HIV, regardless of sexual orientation, as HIV stigma can lead to significant mental health issues, such as low self-esteem, social exclusion and psychological symptoms (Díaz, 2006; Starks et al, 2013).

Studies on ageing and living with HIV seem to have produced varied observations. Research shows that older people with HIV feel that the process of ageing can increase wisdom, tolerance and happiness, but also physical decline, loneliness and lack of support from others (Siegal et al, 1998). However, other studies reveal that older people with HIV experience prejudice, denial and segregation, even though they show resilience to ageism and HIV stigma (Emlet et al, 2011). In a US study of 25 older gay men with HIV, 17 participants believed that they had experienced stigma related to their age and their HIV status, with a further 7 experiencing HIV-related stigma but not ageism (Emlet, 2006).

Methods

The interviews for the present study were conducted during two time periods. First, interviews were carried out in 2011 and 2012 with two of the four informants as part a larger research project focused on HIV, condom use and sexual practices between men (Lee, 2015). Then all four were interviewed during 2020–21. Multiple interviews were conducted with each of the men, with up to four interviews per informant. The data collection was via semi-structured in-depth interviews. Themes were derived from the narratives, reflecting key points or phrases in their stories.

Due to working as a social worker with an AIDS organisation in Hong Kong, the author already had a working relationship with the informants and has maintained contact with them through Grey and Pride, a local organisation for older Chinese *tongzhi*, which is a synonym for lesbian, gay, bisexual, transgender and queer (LGBTQ) in local parlance. While this long relationship has created a bond of trust between the author and informants, the author was concerned that this bond could be in conflict with his researcher role. Therefore, informants were fully apprised of the author's role before informed consents were obtained. This study attempts to understand the social world in which the informants are situated. Warren (2002) refers to the ways each older gay/bisexual man living with HIV assigns meaning to certain facets of their lives and, in turn, attributes such meaning to their lived experiences.

Informants

The four men became aware of their same-sex desires at different stages of their lives, from adolescence to young adulthood. They faced challenges due to being non-heterosexual and learned to live with a stigmatised identity during these early parts of their lives. For instance, if family members or friends found out about their same-sex attraction or behaviours, the men learned how to deal with their reactions (Jones and Hill, 2002). They also experienced living with a stigmatised identity when they learned about their AIDS diagnoses and in their lives with HIV. They shared their experiences of emerging sexuality and living with HIV. To protect their privacy, pseudonyms are used in this chapter.

Wing, aged 77, a self-defined gay man, was born in Hong Kong and is the eldest son in his family. He married in his late twenties and had a child, but the marriage only lasted a few years. After his divorce, Wing took every opportunity to explore his gay life, visiting bathhouses and leaving his parents to look after his child. Due to his Confucian filial duty, he felt that getting married and having offspring had been his only option. Retrospectively, Wing still thinks this route was the only one he could have taken.

Wing was diagnosed with AIDS at 51. Although he had gone through a few serious illnesses associated with HIV, including cytomegalovirus retinitis, Wing remained active, participating in a support network of people living with HIV and gay friends. Wing has not shared his HIV diagnosis with his ex-wife, as they did not have a sexual relationship following their divorce.

Lok, aged 76, is a self-defined gay man who was in a heterosexual marriage. When he was younger, he enjoyed having sex with his wife. Born in China, he came to Hong Kong with his family, in which he is the youngest sibling. He had married in his late twenties, and he had a child from the marriage. Lok said, "If you did not get married and raise a family, relatives would look down on you, saying that you are 'financially incompetent', and this hurts the family's reputation." Lok was active in cruising public toilets and going to gay saunas for sex. He has never had an emotional same-sex relationship; these encounters were all solely sexual. Lok was diagnosed with AIDS when he was 49. His wife was the only person, outside of the hospital and care workers, who knew of his AIDS diagnosis, but she did not know about his sexual experiences with other men.

Keung, aged 75, is a self-defined bisexual man in a heterosexual marriage. He has had sexual relationships with men, although he maintains a sexual and emotional relationship with his wife. He was born in Macao and came to Hong Kong with his family when he was young. Being the only son in the family, remaining unmarried was not an option for him. He married in his late twenties and has children. As a Chinese man, Keung still thought having a family with kids was his only option in life. Keung was very interested in men-only social activities, and this is where he met other gay/bisexual men when he first explored his sexuality. Keung described his non-heterosexuality as being very fluid, but it seems that this has always been affected by social and family pressure. Keung maintained a purely sexual relationship with a man during his early married years, but he ended it since the man wanted a more emotional relationship. Keung was diagnosed with AIDS when he was 53. He was very open about his HIV status, but not his sexuality, with his immediate family, some other relatives and close friends. Keung said, "I brought it [AIDS] all on myself. I can't blame anyone else … I chose this path … maybe it is a part of the script."

Chow, aged 69, is a self-defined bisexual man who is in a heterosexual marriage but has been living separately from his wife since his late twenties. Chow grew up in a village in China. Even though he was sexually interested in men, getting married was the only option for him. He married in his early twenties and became a father. He came to Hong Kong on his own in his late twenties; his wife remained in China with their child. Chow understood that his non-heterosexuality was not a mental illness (as was commonly thought), but he still blamed himself for thinking of men and having sex with them. His attempt to suppress his same-sex desires was very difficult for him, and he wished that he was not interested in men, particularly after being infected with HIV. Chow was diagnosed with AIDS when he was 51, and he was very ashamed of his HIV status. He sometimes wonders if his same-sex desire is a curse for him. Chow did not disclose his AIDS diagnosis to his wife, as he has not had a sexual relationship with her since he left China.

Findings

The four older gay/bisexual men diagnosed with AIDS share similar backgrounds, but also have their own unique constellations of transitional experiences. Focusing on their experiences of sexuality, HIV and ageing, several themes emerged, including 'filiality', 'heterosexist harassment', 'hidden lives' and 'living with ageing'.

Filiality

Same-sex attraction is viewed by some as sinful, immoral or a mental health condition. In many societies, culture is cited as one of the causes of stigmatisation, and this is the case in Hong Kong (Ng and Ma, 2004). The Confucian value of filial piety, which emphasises continuity of lineage, seems to be a major cause of rejection of non-heterosexuality, since it was presumed that there would not be children in same-sex relationships. As a result, many Chinese gay/bisexual men experience prejudice and stigma. Keung considered himself to have a filial responsibility to his parents, especially as the only son in the family:

' "Life is a script", [and] being Chinese, I need to build a family and raise kids ... I am the only child, that's where the pressure comes from. Most of my friends like me [who fancy other men], they are in the same situation, facing enormous pressure from their families ... I was also worried about the pressure from relatives.' (Keung)

Following his Confucian belief, Keung knew that getting married and having children was the only way for him to be accepted as a dutiful son within the Chinese tradition (Lau and Ng, 1989; Kong, 2012). In contrast to the typical Western conceptions of individual and family as separate, individual and family are viewed as a 'unit' in Chinese culture (Chou, 2001). The role of a family member is best understood through the duties the individual owes to their parents, in particular the duties of marriage and 'offspring-production' (9, p 497). The obligation to produce a child is conceptualised in the Confucian principle which bestows responsibility for continuing the bloodline onto each family's male heirs. Apart from pressure from within the immediate family, there is also pressure from other relatives (Liu, 2008).

Lok shared a similar experience and explained further that being unmarried also implies economic failure and that his family would lose face if he could not accomplish his filial duty. He stated:

'It was not only my duty as a son, it was also a way of keeping face. If you don't get married, your relatives will look down on you, thinking that you cannot afford to have a family and wife. It brings shame to my parents. I had to get married.' (Lok)

Keung and Lok described the importance of keeping the connection with immediate family and their network (extended relatives) within the Chinese collectivist culture (Hwang et al, 2003). Staying unmarried was seen as an immoral act by the informants, because it would mean they were unable to fulfil the cultural expectation of filiality. This individualistic action can be considered as conflicting directly with the collective's best interests (Yang, 2007; Yang et al, 2007). As a result, unfulfilled social norms may be thought of as shaming the family rather than just the individual. (Li et al, 2004; Yang and Kleinman, 2008).

Heterosexist harassment

Same-sex desires not only threaten filial piety but also give rise to heterosexism in others. This is despite the fact that male homosexual practices have been well documented in Chinese literature. Certain phrases or terms have been distorted to have negative and hurtful connotations, and these were commonly used in Hong Kong during the period from the 1940s to the 1960s (Wong, 2000). Examples are *kai-dai* (godbrother), which is used to refer to a younger homosexual (Bolton and Hutton, 1995, p 173) or a feminine younger brother, and *si-fat gwai* (asshole), used to refer to men who practise anal intercourse with other men (Chen, 2004, p 140).

Even though none of the informants had disclosed their non-heterosexuality in public or to family members, they still experienced heterosexist harassment in subtle and indirect ways. Chow felt horrified and hurt when he realised the terms *kai-dai* and *si-fat gwai* were undignified terms targeting people with same-sex desires or behaviours. He said:

> 'I did not know what *"kai-dai"* and *"si-fat gwai"* meant until I came to Hong Kong. ... It is horrible ... hurtful ... not all gay men like it [anal sex] ... if people think I like playing backside ... being feminised ... what will they think of me!' (Chow)

This subtle form of heterosexist harassment really upset Chow. He explained that the impact of negative portrayals of gayness meant he was in constant fear of being 'outed' as gay or bisexual. This fear can lead to serious distress (Tucker et al, 2016). In addition, heterosexist harassment is often grounded in the enforcement of traditional gender roles, and effeminate gay/bisexual men are viewed as a violation of normative and acceptable gender behaviour (Herek, 1986). Chow reported how harassment is rooted not only in stereotypes of sexual orientation but also in gender expression. The social constructs of masculinity and gender nonconformity can be a basis for stigma linked to homosexuality, and non-normative gender expression often creates suspicion and disapproval among anti-gay groups. In many situations it can lead to police harassment (Berrill, 1990; Kong, 2010). Chow described his rejection of the general public's attitude towards men who are not masculine enough (see Blashill and Powlishta, 2009; Kong, 2010).

As well as subtle verbal harassment, indirect harassment can also have an impact on individuals. Lok shared a difficult experience in which he heard heterosexist comments from family members: "My sister-in-law used the term *'si-fat gwai'* to joke about her neighbours, and my cousin joined in and [they] laughed at them together. I felt ... angry ... depressed ... because I felt they were laughing at me." Lok was anxious and distressed on hearing those terms, as he associated them with his own same-sex behaviours and desires. Even though the verbal harassment was not directed at him, he was concerned about being identified as a 'disgraced' gay/bisexual man.

Smith and Sharpe (1994) refer to heterosexist harassment as bullying behaviour which is embedded in relations of power and control. For Bonifas (2016), it is repetition and prolonged hostility by a more powerful subject towards a less powerful one that is relevant to the victim's and/or victimiser's perceived or actual sexual identity. Deep down, Wing knew that same-sex desires are not wrong, yet he was not assertive enough to confront harassment.

> 'When people saw two men living together and caring for each other, they called them "*kai-dai*" ... it sounds harmless, but you know when people say it, they are laughing at people like us. It was a derogatory term ... it is awful ... sometimes I wanted to say something, but I did not, because I was scared that they will suspect me [being gay] too, you know.' (Wing)

Wing felt a sense of injustice and anger when hearing heterosexist comments against other gay/bisexual men, but at the same time, he did not have the courage to speak out against it, even though the comments were not directed towards him. The discomfort of being gay within a heterosexist society prevented him from criticising the discriminatory harassment (Leonard et al, 2013).

The narratives presented here illustrate how subtle heterosexism affected the informants, even where they themselves were not being directly targeted (Burn et al, 2005). Also, they show that heterosexist harassment is built on both sexual orientation and gender-related constructs, such as the idea that men should not be effeminate.

Hidden lives

People with same-sex desires and/or HIV share a common ground: their stigmatised identity (or identities) can be concealed through their management of personal information (Crocker et al, 1998). Lok shared how he handled stigma when disclosing his AIDS diagnosis to his wife:

> 'When she [my wife] questioned if I got it [HIV] from sex workers, I just implied that I got it from one [a sex worker] ... I'd rather my wife thinks I got it from sex workers. It is bad enough to be HIV-positive, [but] telling her I had sex with men as a married man? I don't think she could take it.' (Lok)

Keung was in a similar position, and he also chose to make his wife believe that he got HIV from sex workers, not from other men.

> 'My wife was there when the doctor told me my HIV-positive result. She was upset, concerned, she cried ... I wondered if she knew how I got the infection ... but no, my wife thought [and still thinks] it was from sex workers. At least I've led her to think that way.' (Keung)

In the context of HIV/AIDS, stigma often attaches to certain marginalised groups: drug users (Mak et al, 2006); female sex workers and their clients (Wong et al, 2011); and gay/bisexual men (Yeo and Chu, 2017). The informants' choice to hide their same-sex sexual activity be interpreted in different ways. First, the informants may have chosen this option simply because they could, since non-heterosexuality can be concealed. Second, they may have done this because their disclosure of HIV and their sexual history with men might create a 'double stigma' (Grossman, 1991), a conflation of HIV stigma with sexual stigma (Herek, 2009). Third, the choice may have been due to the fact that maintaining or 'passing' (Goffman, 1963) with a heterosexual identity is particularly important to the informants as married men. In China, the wives of gay men are known as *tongqi* (see Tang et al, 2020) or *homowives* (see Kong, 2019). Wang and colleagues (2020) report that the impact of stigma on gay men's wives is detrimental, with many wives experiencing serious mental and physical health problems as well as threats on their lives.

Negative attitudes towards people living with HIV within the gay community have been documented since the beginning of the epidemic (Epstein, 1996). HIV-related stigma causes high levels of anxiety, loneliness and depressive symptoms among HIV-positive gay/bisexual men (Courtenay-Quirk et al, 2006; Smit et al, 2012). One way this has been expressed is the reaction to lipodystrophy. This is a condition where fat tissue is redistributed abnormally within the body, resulting in, for example, flattening or indentation of convex contours of the face. The impact of lipodystrophy on gay/bisexual men with HIV is discussed in the literature on gay ageing as well as the literature on HIV. Lipodystrophy is also referred to as 'the look of AIDS', and it can add an additional level of stigma from within the gay community (Gorman and Nelson, 2004, p 81). Collins et al (2000) report that lipodystrophy can negatively affect self-esteem and self-image, create problems with social or sexual relations, threaten locus of control and force HIV disclosure. Lok started visiting gay saunas in Hong Kong when his general health improved, but he developed minor lipodystrophy on his face when he first started HIV treatment, causing him to worry abut the reaction he might get: "With the sign of my face, I was worried that people may guess [I have AIDS] and spread rumours around ... you know they [gay men] can be quite gossipy."

Living with ageing

Ageing may bring some additional and significant challenges for gay/bisexual men living with HIV. All the informants were diagnosed with AIDS in mid to late life. Due to their HIV status and associated health conditions, the diagnosis deterred them from connecting with the gay/bisexual scene for some time. Two informants disconnected from the scene completely, and two eventually reconnected with it. Wing and Lok continued to visit saunas after their diagnoses, but both were also aware of ageism in Hong Kong. Wing said: "I started going to gay saunas in Hong Kong when my health improved, but I only go to those saunas that are friendly for older men ... in fact, I would rather go to gay saunas in Shenzhen (China), as younger gays are more elder-friendly." Lok also rejoined the gay/bisexual scene, primarily for sex. He was aware that most of the gay/bisexual scenes in Hong Kong preferred men who are young and have certain body types.

> 'Most saunas only welcome young and good-looking guys. During the last eight or nine years, I only went to the sauna where mostly older and mature men go – for example, Sauna K in Hong Kong. ... Why? I feel more comfortable there. At least I won't be looked down on by them [younger gays].' (Lok)

Wing and Lok were conscious of the ageism that existed and chose elder-friendly sexual venues where they felt more accepted and less likely to experience personal stigma (Steward et al, 2008), as they were aware that the majority of gay culture places emphasis on youth (Robinson, 2011).

In contrast, Chow and Keung have not experienced gay-related ageism since they stopped visiting the gay/bisexual scene. In fact, they stopped having sex with other men because of concern for their weakened immune system and the possibility of passing the HIV virus to others. When these two informants were asked if they felt lonely or isolated and not connected to other gay/bisexual men, Chow stated:

> 'The nurses in the [AIDS] clinic say our immune systems are weaker than people without HIV. Also, I don't want to infect other people. ... Why? Even though we only kiss, or caress each other, or I perform oral sex on them (I don't let other people suck me, especially since most people do not want to put a condom on for oral sex), still the psychological stress is there ... and ... anyway, it was only sex, even without HIV, I would not go because I do not need it as much as when I was younger. I am okay with it.' (Chow)

Keung similarly described his reluctance to be involved in the sex scene within the gay community.

> 'Apart from the health issue – my immune system is weaker than average for men of my age – I would feel very guilty if I passed the virus to someone by accident. Yes, I still fancy men, but ... I don't feel lonely ... I have a family, a wife, someone to go home to.' (Keung)

Chow and Keung did not have personal experience of ageism within the gay community because they avoided contact with the community after their HIV diagnosis. Apart from concern for their weakened immune systems, these men wanted to avoid passing HIV on to others, which would cause them to feel guilt, even if it were to happen when practising safe sex (Keogh et al, 1998; Hamann et al, 2017).

On one hand, Chow's comment on sex – "I do not need it" – and Keung's comment on loneliness – "I don't feel lonely" – could be interpreted as their experiences of ageing not being dominated by loneliness or exclusion on account of ageism towards older gay/bisexual men (Hostetler, 2004). On the other hand, their withdrawal from sex with men completely may be due to internalised stigma related to their HIV status (Herek et al, 2009; Chan et al, 2021), especially in light of their background stories and their ongoing sexual interest in men.

Discussion

Due to the small sample size and the informants having similar characteristics, the findings do not represent a universal position. However, the information-rich narratives of four older gay/bisexual provide valuable insight. These narratives indicate that the men's lived experiences during a time of severe criminal and social sanctions as well as the AIDS epidemic, along with their long-term illness, have influenced the way they live their lives in the Hong Kong context. Their narratives demonstrate how heterosexism, HIV stigma and ageism have influenced their lives. The following discussion links these themes with existing literature and shows some comparable themes.

First, the informants experienced psychological heterosexism due to subtle and indirect heterosexist comments. This is in line with research in some European societies that found older LGBTQ individuals are on the receiving end of peers' prejudice, heterosexist harassment and even homophobic bullying (Meisner and Hynie, 2009; Cook-Daniels and Munson, 2010; Bonifas, 2016). In addition, the use of subtle and indirect terms to degrade older gay/bisexual men is not exclusive to Chinese culture. In a study from the United States, Johnson and colleagues (2005) found that older LGBTQ individuals in care face subtle or overt discriminatory attitudes by staff and other residents.

Second, the manifestation of cultural heterosexism at an institutional level and subsequent omission or invisibility of older gay/bisexual men in receipt of care or support has also been found in previous studies (Leonard et al, 2013; Orel and Fruhauf, 2015; Bonifas, 2016). Heteronormative culture forces many gay/bisexual men to conceal their sexual orientation (Van den Berg, 2016) or even return to the closet when they are in institutional settings (see Schwinn and Dinkel, 2015, on this issue in long-term care).

Hong Kong currently lacks any anti-discrimination legislation for sexual minorities, so sexual minorities are exposed to a heterosexist culture without any protection (Chan, 2005); this exposure creates a significant risk to their mental health (Kwok and Wu, 2015). It is likely that older Chinese gay/bisexual men suffer from stress due to being in a minority, as has been found in studies of older LGBTQ in other parts of the world (Kuyper and Fokkema, 2010; Gonçalves et al, 2020).

Third, the impact of heteronormativity affects not only older married Chinese gay/bisexual men but also their wives. Even though research suggests that gay/bisexual men's wives are more of a phenomenon in China than in Hong Kong (see Kong, 2019; Tang et al, 2020), their existence in both places seems to be influenced by heterosexist culture combined with an ideology that stresses filiality (Huang et al, 2020). The connection between heteronormative culture and Confucian filial beliefs are also found in other studies (Zhou, 2006; Wong and Poon, 2013; Hua et al, 2019).

Fourth, stigma management was evident among the older Chinese gay/bisexual men in this study in relation to both sexual orientation and HIV status. For example, to reduce the risk of stigma, they hid their HIV status within the gay community and they implied that their HIV infection came from sex workers rather than sex with other men. The use of stigma management to adapt to oppressive situations has been shown in studies of HIV attitudes within the gay community (Chenard, 2007) and outside the gay community (Hammond, 2015; Weitzer, 2018). The stigma management strategies found in this study were in line with findings from studies on HIV-positive older gay/bisexual men in other countries (Siegel et al, 1998; Courtenay-Quirk et al, 2006; Makoae et al, 2008).

Fifth, the term 'double stigma' reflects the combined impact of heterosexism and HIV stigma. This was a driver for Wing and Lok to lie about the mode of transmission being from sex workers rather than from other gay/bisexual men. Double stigma can become internalised (Herek et al, 2009). For instance, Keung believed "having AIDS is a part of the script [I fancy men]". Chow regretted his same-sex desires, believing his AIDS diagnosis is payback for having sex with men; this belief indicates that his internalised HIV stigma has had a re-traumatising effect in relation to his perception of his own sexuality. Both these informants internalised the stigma about male homosexuality (Meyer, 2003) coupled with stigma about HIV; this narrative is in line with studies in Chinese societies (Xu et al, 2017; Liu et al, 2021) as well as those focusing on Western cultures (Overstreet et al, 2013; Boone et al, 2016).

Sixth, apart from the double stigma of sexual orientation and HIV, older gay/bisexual men with or without HIV also face the double stigma of 'being gay in a world of heterosexual supremacy, being old in a LGB community that values youth' (Haber, 2009, p 277). Older gay/bisexual men with HIV are susceptible to stigma related to both age and HIV status within the gay community (Lyons et al, 2015). In the present study, two of the informants choose to avoid mainstream youth-orientated gay scenes, whereas the other two chose to avoid the gay scene completely. Even though their strategies can be understood as following a normative social code to avoid stigma enactments (Herek, 2009), they can also be interpreted as internalised ageism (Slater et al, 2013; Wight et al, 2015) which incorporates negative social stereotypes about ageing as a part of self-identification (Emlet, 2006; Slater et al, 2013).

Conclusion

This chapter has demonstrated that older Chinese gay/bisexual men living with HIV in Hong Kong encounter multiple experiences of stigma related to their sexual orientation, HIV status and ageing, and these are experienced intersectionally and at individual and institutional levels. The author has witnessed how stigma can be damaging for people generally, and this is particularly true for older non-heterosexual men with HIV living in a society that does not consider it necessary to provide protection or respect for sexual minorities.

The accounts of the men who took part in this study illustrate how Confucianism, especially its emphasis on filiality, reinforces heteronormativity. This emphasis creates an environment where the men may find it difficult or even impossible to imagine having a relationship or finding love with a person of the same sex, thus reinforcing the internalised stigma of being a gay/bisexual man. The Confucian concept of 'losing face', not only for oneself but also for one's family only serves to reinforce the non-negotiable social contract of marriage. A path of divergence from filial piety serves to make the gay/bisexual man susceptible not only to suffering psychological distress, but also to enduring social stigmatisation and cultural trauma that this marginalised population may encounter within the context of Chinese Confucian society.

The findings suggest that older Chinese gay/bisexual men with HIV remain invisible and closeted, affected by the barriers caused by heterosexism, HIV stigma and ageism that inhibit successful ageing both within and outside the gay community. What we can learn from the stories and lived experiences of these men is, first, that their experiences and voices can enhance and enrich our understanding of other older gay/bisexual men with HIV, who might encounter similar situations. Second, to provide culturally appropriate interventions, mental health services targeting this marginalised population should address socioecological issues, such as social distress specific to the ideology of heterosexual marriage within a heteronormative culture. Third, we can respond to the needs of this vulnerable and marginalised group by providing community-based interventions, such as self-help groups or charitable organisations that can provide programmes that address their needs and empower individuals to rebuild their support networks. Fourth, we can pave the way for further research and for social services to be developed so that the unheard voices and unmet needs of this forgotten section of society can be heard and addressed.

References

Atchley, R.C. and Barusch, A.S. (eds) (2004) *Social Forces and Aging: An Introduction to Social Gerontology* (10th edn), Belmont, CA: Wadsworth/ Thompson Learning.

Balzarini, R.N., Shumlich, E.J., Kohut, T. and Campbell, L. (2018) 'Dimming the "halo" around monogamy: re-assessing stigma surrounding consensually non-monogamous romantic relationships as a function of personal relationship orientation', *Frontiers in Psychology*, 9(894): 1–13.

Berrill, K.T. (1990) 'Anti-gay violence and victimization in the United States: an overview', *Journal of Interpersonal Violence*, 5(3): 274–94.

Blashill, A.J. and Powlishta, K.K. (2009) 'Gay stereotypes: the use of sexual orientation as a cue for gender-related attributes', *Sex Roles*, 61(11): 783–93.

Bolton, K. and Hutton, C. (1995) 'Bad and banned language: triad secret societies, the censorship of the Cantonese vernacular, and colonial language policy in Hong Kong', *Language in Society*, 24(2): 159–86.

Bonifas, R.P. (2016) 'The prevalence of elder bullying and impact on LGBT elders', in D.A. Harley and P.B. Teaster (eds) *Handbook of LGBT Elders*, Cham, Switzerland: Springer, pp 359–72.

Boone, M.R., Cook, S.H. and Wilson, P.A. (2016) 'Sexual identity and HIV status influence the relationship between internalized stigma and psychological distress in Black gay and bisexual men', *AIDS Care*, 28(6): 764–70.

Burn, S.M., Kadlec, K. and Rexer, R. (2005) 'Effects of subtle heterosexism on gays, lesbians, and bisexuals', *Journal of Homosexuality*, 49(2): 23–38.

Chan, P.C. (2005) 'The lack of sexual orientation anti-discrimination legislation in Hong Kong: breach of international and domestic legal obligations', *The International Journal of Human Rights*, 9(1): 69–106.

Chan, R.C.H., Mak, W.W., Ma, G.Y. and Cheung, M. (2021) 'Interpersonal and intrapersonal manifestations of HIV stigma and their impacts on psychological distress and life satisfaction among people living with HIV: toward a dual-process model', *Quality of Life Research*, 30(1): 145–56.

Chen, C. (2004) 'On the Hong Kong Chinese subtitling of English swearwords', *Meta: Translators' Journal*, 49(1): 135–47.

Chenard, C. (2007) 'The impact of stigma on the self-care behaviors of HIV-positive gay men striving for normalcy', *Journal of the Association of Nurses in AIDS Care*, 18(3): 23–32.

Chou, W.-S. (2000) *Tongzhi: Politics of Same-Sex Eroticism in Chinese Societies*, New York: Haworth.

Chou, W.-S. (2001) 'Homosexuality and the cultural politics of *tongzhi* in Chinese societies', *Journal of Homosexuality*, 40(3–4): 27–46.

Collins, E., Wagner, C. and Walmsley, S. (2000) 'Psychosocial impact of the lipodystrophy syndrome in HIV infection', *AIDS Reader New York*, 10(9): 546–51.

Cook-Daniels, L. and Munson, M. (2010) 'Sexual violence, elder abuse, and sexuality of transgender adults, age 50: results of three surveys', *Journal of GLBT Family Studies*, 6(2): 142–77.

Courtenay-Quirk, C., Wolitski, R.J., Parsons, J.T., Gomez, C.A. and Seropositive Urban Men's Study Team (2006) 'Is HIV/AIDS stigma dividing the gay community? Perceptions of HIV-positive men who have sex with men', *AIDS Education and Prevention*, 18(1): 56–67.

Crocker, J., Major, B. and Steele, C. (1998) 'Social stigma', in D.T. Gilbert, S.T. Fiske and G. Lindzey (eds) *The Handbook of Social Psychology*, Vol 2 (4th edn), New York: McGraw-Hill, pp 504–53.

Díaz, R.M. (2006) 'In our own backyard: HIV/AIDS stigmatization in the Latino gay community', in N. Teunis and G. Herdt (eds) *Sexual Inequalities and Social Justice*, Berkeley: University of California Press, pp 50–65.

Dong, X. and Xu, Y. (2016) 'Filial piety among global Chinese adult children: a systematic review', *Research and Review: Journal of Social Science*, 2(1): 46–55.

Emlet, C.A. (2006) '"You're awfully old to have this disease": experiences of stigma and ageism in adults 50 years and older living with HIV/AIDS', *The Gerontologist*, 46(6): 781–90.

Emlet, C.A., Tozay, S. and Raveis, V.H. (2011) '"I'm not going to die from the AIDS": resilience in aging with HIV disease', *The Gerontologist*, 51(1): 101–11.

Epstein, S. (1996) *Impure Science: AIDS, Activism, and the Politics of Knowledge*, Berkeley: University of California Press.

Flowers, P., Duncan, B. and Frankis, J. (2000) 'Community, responsibility and culpability: HIV risk-management amongst Scottish gay men', *Journal of Community and Applied Social Psychology*, 10(4): 285–300.

Gewirtz-Meydan, A., Hafford-Letchfield, T., Benyamini, Y., Phelan, A., Jackson, J. and Ayalon, L. (2018) Ageism and sexuality, in L. Ayalon and C. Tesch-Römer (eds) *Contemporary Perspectives on Ageism*, New York: Springer, pp 149–62.

Goffman, E. (1963) *Stigma: Notes on the Management of a Spoiled Identity*, New York: Simon and Schuster.

Gonçalves, J.A.R., Costa, P.A. and Leal, I. (2020) 'Minority stress in older Portuguese gay and bisexual men and its impact on sexual and relationship satisfaction', *Sexuality Research and Social Policy*, 17(2): 209–18.

Gorman, E.M. and Nelson, K. (2004) 'From a far place: social and cultural considerations about HIV among midlife and older gay men', in G. Herdt and B. de Vries (eds) *Gay and Lesbian Aging: Research and Future Directions*, pp 73–93.

Grossman, A.H. (1991) 'Gay men and HIV/AIDS: understanding the double stigma', *Journal of the Association of Nurses in AIDS Care*, 2(4): 28–32.

Haber, D. (2009) 'Gay aging', *Gerontology and Geriatrics Education*, 30(3): 267–80.

Hamann, C., Pizzinato, A., Weber, J.L.A. and Rocha, K.B. (2017) 'Narratives about risk and guilt among patients of a specialized HIV infection service: implications for care in sexual health', *Saúde e Sociedade*, 26(3): 651–63.

Hammond, N. (2015) 'Men who pay for sex and the sex work movement: client responses to stigma and increased regulation of commercial sex policy', *Social Policy and Society*, 14(1): 93–102.

Heaphy, B., Yip, A.K.T. and Thompson, D. (2003) *Lesbian, Gay and Bisexual Lives over 50: Report on the Project: 'The Social and Policy Implications of Non-Heterosexual Ageing'*, Nottingham, UK: York House Publications.

Herek, G.M. (1986) 'On heterosexual masculinity: some psychical consequences of the social construction of gender and sexuality', *American Behavioral Scientist*, 29(5): 563–77.

Herek, G.M. (1990) 'The context of anti-gay violence: notes on cultural and psychological heterosexism', *Journal of Interpersonal Violence*, 5(3): 316–33.

Herek, G.M. (1995) 'Psychological heterosexism in the United States: lesbian, gay, and bisexual identities over the lifespan', in A.R. D'Augelli and C.J. Patterson (eds) *Lesbian Gay and Bisexual Identities over the Lifespan: Psychological Perspectives*, Oxford: Oxford University Press, pp 321–46.

Herek, G.M. (1996) 'Heterosexism and homophobia', in R.P. Cabaj and T.S. Stein (eds) *Textbook of Homosexuality and Mental Health*, Washington, DC: American Psychiatric Press:, pp 101–13.

Herek, G.M. (2009) 'Sexual stigma and sexual prejudice in the United States: A conceptual framework', in D.A. Hope (ed) *Contemporary Perspectives on Lesbian, Gay and Bisexual Identities: The 54th Nebraska Symposium on Motivation*, New York: Springer, pp 65–111.

Herek, G.M., Gillis, J.R. and Cogan, J.C. (2009) 'Internalized stigma among sexual minority adults: insights from a social psychological perspective', *Journal of Counseling Psychology*, 56(1): 32–43.

Heyward, W.L. and Curran, J.W. (1988) 'The epidemiology of AIDS in the US', *Scientific American*, 259(4): 72–81.

Hinsch, B. (1990) *Passion of the Cut Sleeve: The Male Homosexual Tradition in China*, Los Angeles: University of California Press.

Ho, P.S. (1995) 'Male homosexual identity in Hong Kong', *Journal of Homosexuality*, 29(1): 71–88.

Hostetler, A.J. (2004) 'Old, gay, and alone? The ecology of well-being among middle-aged and older single gay men', in B. DeVries and G. Herdt (eds) *Gay and Lesbian Aging and Research: Future Directions*, New York: Springer, pp 143–76.

Hua, B., Yang, V.F. and Goldsen, K.F. (2019) 'LGBT older adults at a crossroads in mainland China: the intersections of stigma, cultural values, and structural changes within a shifting context', *The International Journal of Aging and Human Development*, 88(4): 440–56.

Huang, Y.T., Chan, R.C.H. and Cui, L. (2020) 'Filial piety, internalized homonegativity, and depressive symptoms among Taiwanese gay and bisexual men: a mediation analysis', *American Journal of Orthopsychiatry*, 90(3): 340–9.

Hwang, A., Francesco, A.M. and Kessler, E. (2003) 'The relationship between individualism-collectivism, face, and feedback and learning processes in Hong Kong, Singapore, and the United States', *Journal of Cross-Cultural Psychology*, 34(1): 72–91.

Johnson, M.J., Jackson, N.C., Arnette, J.K. and Koffman, S.D. (2005) 'Gay and lesbian perceptions of discrimination in retirement care facilities', *Journal of Homosexuality*, 49(2): 83–102.

Jones, B.E. and Hill, M.J. (2002) *Mental Health Issues in Lesbian, Gay, Bisexual and Transgender Communities*, Washington, DC: American Psychiatric Publishing Inc.

Keogh, P., Peardsell, S., Davies, P., Hickson, F. and Weatherburn, P. (1998) 'Gay men and HIV: community responses and personal risks', *Journal of Psychology and Human Sexuality*, 10(3–4): 59–73.

Kong, T.S.K. (2010) *Chinese Male Homosexualities: Memba, Tongzhi and Golden Boy*, Abingdon, UK: Routledge.

Kong, T.S.K. (2012) 'A fading *tongzhi* heterotopia: Hong Kong older gay men's use of spaces', *Sexualities*, 15(8): 896–916.

Kong, T.S.K. (2019) *Oral Histories of Older Gay Men in Hong Kong: Unspoken but Unforgotten*, Hong Kong: Hong Kong University Press.

Kutner, B.A., Simoni, J.M., Aunon, F.M., Creegan, E. and Balán, I.C. (2020) 'How stigma toward anal sexuality promotes concealment and impedes health-seeking behavior in the US among cisgender men who have sex with men', *Archives of Sexual Behavior*, 50(4): 1651–63.

Kuyper, L. and Fokkema, C.M. (2010) 'Loneliness among older lesbian, gay, and bisexual adults: the role of minority stress', *Archives of Sexual Behavior*, 39(5): 1171–80.

Kwok, D.K. and Wu, J. (2015) 'Chinese attitudes towards sexual minorities in Hong Kong: implications for mental health', *International Review of Psychiatry*, 27(5): 444–54.

Lau, M.P. and Ng, M.L. (1989) 'Homosexuality in Chinese culture', *Culture, Medicine and Psychiatry*, 13: 465–88.

Leask, C., Elford, J., Bor, R., Miller, R. and Johnson, M. (1997) 'Selective disclosure: a pilot investigation into changes in family relationships since HIV diagnosis', *Journal of Family Therapy*, 19(1): 59–69.

Lee, M.W.B. (2015) *Sexual Acts, Masculinities and Condom Use among Hong Kong Chinese Men Who Have Sex with Men (MSM)*, PhD thesis, University of Hong Kong.

Leonard, W., Duncan, D. and Barrett, C. (2013) 'What a difference a gay makes: the constitution of the "older gay man"', in A. Kampf, B.L. Marshall and A. Petersen (eds) *Aging Men, Masculinities and Modern Medicine*, London: Routledge, pp 105–20.

Li, J., Wang, L. and Fischer, K.W. (2004) 'The organisation of Chinese shame concepts', *Cognition and Emotion*, 18(6): 767–97.

Liu, D. (2003) *History of Erotica in China*, Yinchuan, China: Ningxia People's Press.

Liu, F. (2008) 'Negotiating the filial self: young-adult only-children and intergenerational relationships in China', *Young*, 16(4): 409–30.

Liu, F., Chui, H. and Chung, M.C. (2021) 'The moderating effect of filial piety on the relationship between perceived public stigma and internalized homophobia: a national survey of the Chinese LGB population', *Sexuality Research and Social Policy*, 18(1): 160–9.

Lu, T.L.D. (2009) 'Heritage conservation in post-colonial Hong Kong', *International Journal of Heritage Studies*, 15(2–3): 258–72.

Lyons, A., Croy, S., Barrett, C. and Whyte, C. (2015) 'Growing old as a gay man: how life has changed for the gay liberation generation', *Ageing and Society*, 35(10): 2229–50.

Mak, W.W., Mo, P.K., Cheung, R.Y., Woo, J., Cheung, F.M. and Lee, D. (2006) 'Comparative stigma of HIV/AIDS, SARS, and tuberculosis in Hong Kong', *Social Science & Medicine*, 63(7): 1912–22.

Makoae, L.N., Greeff, M., Phetlhu, R.D., Uys, L.R., Naidoo, J.R., Kohi, T.W. and Holzemer, W.L. (2008) 'Coping with HIV-related stigma in five African countries', *Journal of the Association of Nurses in AIDS Care*, 19(2): 137–46.

Meisner, B.A. and Hynie, M. (2009) 'Ageism with heterosexism: self-perceptions, identity, and psychological health in older gay and lesbian adults', *Gay and Lesbian Issues and Psychology Review*, 5(1): 51–8.

Meyer, I.H. (2003) 'Prejudice, social stress, and mental health in lesbian, gay, and bisexual populations: conceptual issues and research evidence', *Psychological Bulletin*, 129(5): 674–97.

Ng, M.L. and Ma, J.L.C. (2004) 'Sexuality in Hong Kong Special Administrative Region of the People's Republic of China', in B. Francoeur and R.J. Noonan (eds) *The Continuum Complete International Encyclopedia of Sexuality*, New York: Continuum Publishing Group, Ltd.

Orel, N.A. and Fruhauf, C.A. (2015) 'The intersection of culture, family, and individual aspects: a guiding model for LGBT older adults', in N.A. Orel and C.A. Fruhauf (eds) *The Lives of LGBT Older Adults: Understanding Challenges and Resilience*, Washington, DC: American Psychological Association, pp 3–24.

Overstreet, N.M., Earnshaw, V.A., Kalichman, S.C. and Quinn, D.M. (2013) 'Internalized stigma and HIV status disclosure among HIV-positive Black men who have sex with men', *AIDS Care*, 25(4): 466–71.

Quinn, D.M. and Earnshaw, V.A. (2011) 'Understanding concealable stigmatized identities: the role of identity in psychological, physical, and behavioral outcomes', *Social Issues and Policy Review*, 5(1): 160–90.

Robinson, P. (2011) 'The influence of ageism on relations between old and young gay men', in Y. Smaal and G. Willett (eds) *Out Here: Gay and Lesbian Perspectives VI*, Clayton, Australia: Monash University Publishing, pp 188–200.

Ruan, F.F. (1991) *Sex in China: Studies of Sexology in Chinese Culture*, New York: Plenum.

Schwinn, S.V. and Dinkel, S.A. (2015) 'Changing the culture of long-term care: combating heterosexism', *Online Journal of Issues in Nursing*, 20: 2. doi: 10.3912/OJIN.Vol20No02PPT03

Sheon, N. and Crosby, G.M. (2004) 'Ambivalent tales of HIV disclosure in San Francisco', *Social Science & Medicine*, 58(11): 2105–18.

Shields, S.A. and Harriman, R.E. (1984) 'Fear of male homosexuality: cardiac responses of low and high homonegative males', *Journal of Homosexuality*, 10(1–2): 53–67.

Siegel, K., Lune, H. and Meyer, I.H. (1998) 'Stigma management among gay/bisexual men with HIV/AIDS', *Qualitative Sociology*, 21(1): 3–24.

Silverschanz, P., Cortina, L.M., Konik, J. and Magley, V.J. (2008) 'Slurs, snubs, and queer jokes: incidence and impact of heterosexist harassment in academia', *Sex Roles*, 58(3–4): 179–91.

Slater, L.Z., Moneyham, L., Vance, D.E., Raper, J.L., Mugavero, M.J. and Childs, G. (2013) 'Support, stigma, health, coping, and quality of life in older gay men with HIV', *Journal of Association of Nurses in AIDS Care*, 24(1): 38–49.

Slevin, K.F. and Linneman, T.J. (2010) 'Old gay men's bodies and masculinities', *Men and Masculinities*, 12(4): 483–507.

Smit, P.J., Brady, M., Carter, M., Fernandes, R., Lamore, L., Meulbroek, M. and Thompson, M. (2012) 'HIV-related stigma within communities of gay men: a literature review', *AIDS Care*, 24(4): 405–12.

Smith, P. and Sharp, S. (eds) (1994) *School Bullying: Insights and Perspectives*, London: Routledge.

Starks, T.J., Rendina, H.J., Breslow, A.S., Parsons, J.T. and Golub, S.A. (2013) 'The psychological cost of anticipating HIV stigma for HIV-negative gay and bisexual men', *AIDS and Behavior*, 17(8): 2732–41.

Steward, W.T., Herek, G.M., Ramakrishna, J., Bharat, S, Chandy, S., Wrubel, J. and Ekstrand, M.L. (2008) 'HIV-related stigma: adapting a theoretical framework for use in India', *Social Science & Medicine*, 67(8): 1225–35.

Suen, Y.T. (2017) 'Older single gay men's body talk: resisting and rigidifying the aging discourse in the gay community', *Journal of Homosexuality*, 64(3): 397–414.

Tang, L., Meadows, C. and Li, H. (2020) 'How gay men's wives in China practice co-cultural communication: culture, identity, and sensemaking', *Journal of International and Intercultural Communication*, 13(1): 13–31.

Tucker, J.S., Ewing, B.A., Espelage, D.L., Green, H.D., Jr, de la Haye, K. and Pollard, M.S. (2016) 'Longitudinal associations of homophobic name-calling victimization with psychological distress and alcohol use during adolescence', *Journal of Adolescent Health*, 59(1): 110–15.

Van den Berg, E. (2016) '"The closet": a dangerous heteronormative space', *South African Review of Sociology*, 47(3): 25–43.

Wang, Y., Wilson, A., Chen, R., Hu, Z., Peng, K. and Xu, S. (2020) 'Behind the rainbow, "Tongqi" wives of men who have sex with men in China: a systematic review', *Frontiers in Psychology* [online], 10: 2929. doi: 10.3389/fpsyg.2019.02929

Warren, C.A.B. (2002) 'Qualitative interviewing', in J.F. Gubrium and J.A. Holstein (eds) *Handbook of Interview Research: Context and Method*, Thousand Oaks, CA: Sage, pp 83–102.

Weinberg, G. (1972) *Society and the Healthy Homosexual*, New York: St. Martin's.

Weitzer, R. (2018) 'Resistance to sex work stigma', *Sexualities*, 21(5–6): 717–29.

Wight, R.G., LeBlanc, A.J., Meyer, I.H. and Harig, F.A. (2015) 'Internalized gay ageism, mattering, and depressive symptoms among midlife and older gay-identified men', *Social Science & Medicine*, 147: 200–8.

Wong, C.C. (2000) 'Sworn brotherhood: an analysis from a historical perspective of 'sun ba gets fortune by saving man', *Hanxue Yanjiu*, 18(2): 163–85.

Wong, J.P.H. and Poon, M.K.L. (2013) 'Challenginf homophobia and heterosexism through storytelling and critical dialogue among Hong Kong Chinese immigrant parents in Toronto', *Culture, Health and Sexuality*, 15(1): 15–28.

Wong, W.C., Holroyd, E. and Bingham, A. (2011) 'Stigma and sex work from the perspective of female sex workers in Hong Kong', *Sociology of Health and Illness*, 33(1): 50–65.

Woody, I. (2014) 'Aging out: a qualitative exploration of ageism and heterosexism among aging African American lesbians and gay men', *Journal of Homosexuality*, 61(1): 145–65.

Xu, X., Sheng, Y., Khoshnood, K. and Clark, K. (2017) 'Factors predicting internalized stigma among men who have sex with men living with HIV in Beijing, China', *Journal of the Association of Nurses in AIDS Care*, 28(1): 142–53.

Yang, L.H. (2007) 'Application of mental illness stigma theory to Chinese societies: synthesis and new directions', *Singapore Medical Journal*, 48(11): 977–85.

Yang, L.H. and Kleinman, A. (2008) '"Face" and the embodiment of stigma in China: the cases of schizophrenia and AIDS', *Social Science & Medicine*, 67(3): 398–408.

Yang, L.H, Kleinman, A., Link, B.G., Phelan, J.C., Lee, S. and Good, B. (2007) 'Culture and stigma: adding moral experience to stigma theory', *Social Science & Medicine*, 64(7): 1524–35.

Yeo, T.E.D. and Chu, T.H. (2017) 'Social-cultural factors of HIV-related stigma among the Chinese general population in Hong Kong', *AIDS Care*, 29(10): 1255–9.

Zhou, Y.R. (2006) 'Homosexuality, seropositivity and family obligations: perspectives of HIV-infected men who have sex with men in China', *Culture, Health and Sexuality*, 8(6): 487–500.

PART III

Intersectional lives, multiple stigmas

8

Out in Africa: facing the HIV other in Nairobi

Casey Charles

Losing self, facing others

In 2009, I came to Kenya to write poetry, having received a partial grant to attend Summer Literary Seminars, a writing workshop sponsored by Concordia University in Canada. I was trying to remake myself, trying to transition from literary critic to creative writer. The location of the seminar seemed 'exotic' – I had friends in Nairobi, a sister in Tanzania – but my main focus was craft, finding my voice. What transpired during my stay was entirely unanticipated for a 50-something gay professor from Montana who was quietly managing his HIV. In the process of discovering myself as a writer, I confronted the core of my identity through a face-to-face encounter with the other, with the otherness of HIV in Nairobi – an engagement, an intersection with the melancholy and vulnerability of other long-term HIV survivors (HIVLTS) whose stories were deeply uncanny, both shared and unknown.[1] Through recounting their stories, through losing myself in relating the narratives of a heterosexual ex-sex worker from East Africa and others, I realised how my sexuality produced an unlikely tie to the other.

While it is impossible to ascribe my extraordinary contact with AIDS in East Africa specifically to the pleasure of self-loss or the relinquishment of ego, there remains a dynamic in the process of understanding (that is, *standing under*) another – some intimacy in the pleasure of telling another's story – that corresponds deeply to the trajectory of death and life of an HIVLTS. My receptivity to the gestalt of understanding is arguably ascribable in part to the position of the gay HIV subject, who often has experienced the surrender of ego in the process of sexuality. Many years ago, Leo Bersani's famous polemic declared that sex between men – and particularly that passive anal intercourse that frequently transmitted HIV – was not a springboard for a queer cultural revolution but, on the contrary, a reminder that sex at its core

---

[1] Levinas' concept of 'facing' is explored in Butler (2004). I base my interview encounters with HIVLTS on the concept of facing the other.

involves a disintegration, 'a *losing sight* of the self' in *jouissance*. For Bersani, the AIDS pandemic and its killing of sexual subjects around the world illustrates that sex between men often partakes of the invaluable experience of powerlessness, loss of ego, relinquishment of dominance (1987, p 222).[2]

For those of us who have so far survived the perils of AIDS, those of us who lost sight of ourselves but are still surviving well into the 21st century, Bersani's speculation, based in part on the insistence of psychoanalysis on the nonsense of the drive, continues to resonate not just sexually, but socially and psychologically.[3] As long-term survivors, many of us have had our death sentences commuted by highly active antiretroviral therapy (HAART), and many of us have overcome the stigma of contamination to enter the brave new world of pre-exposure prophylaxis (PrEP) and undetectable barebacking.[4] But if sex for some of us is no longer lethal, and a full lifespan is for many of us within grasp, the reality of a *losing sight of self* not only continues to haunt us as survivors but also looms on the horizon with the more universal predicament of age.

Within the intricacies of this context – fraught with guilt and promise, with loss and gain – my own lost self found a kind of intimacy, almost serendipitously, through a detour into the world of HIV during my attendance at a Nairobi writers' workshop. That detour led to this account of my experience, one that comes not without serious misgivings about my ability to represent the precarious lives of others whose social and cultural contexts are in many ways beyond my epistemological grasp. Faced with gender, class, racial and even global divides, my essay about other HIVLTS in Nairobi not only borders on cultural appropriation but also raises philosophical questions about the value and validity of my recounting of any encounter with the other. 'Is it possible, and how is it possible, for … men [to] research women, white people, people of color, or vice versa?' ask Fawcett and Hearn in their essay about the pitfalls of social research (2004, p 202). In my case, despite the intersection of HIV positivity – of blood tests, drug regiments, opportunistic infections, dead friends, stigma – I still struggle to overcome the structural obstacles faced by a White man from the West, an upper-middle-class, cisgender professor and writer seeking to transmit and illustrate (and, at worst, capitalise on) the narratives of others

---

[2] Since the start of the pandemic, 34.7 million people have died of AIDS, now in its fifth decade (UNAIDS, nd).

[3] The drive derives perverse pleasure from desire's impossible quest for fulfilment, according to the psychoanalytic tradition Bersani employs in his argument (Johnston, 2018).

[4] HAART refers to the drug combinations currently used to impede activity of the virus. PrEP most commonly involves the ingestion of Truvada, a two-drug combination that prevents transmission and is commonly taken by sexually active negative partners.

he does not know beyond an interview or support group (Jackson, 2021). What authority or capacity have I to write about others?

The subject of research is always, at some level, other to the researcher, Fawcett and Hearn conclude (2004). Into this epistemological dilemma, solipsistic as it can ultimately become theoretically, arrived a naive poet to a workshop in Africa in 2009, at the outset uninterested in the happenstance that had brought him to one of the densest HIV populations on the globe. Into this 'Third World' came a 'First World' privileged queer man, swallowing antiretrovirals (ARTs) on an empty stomach to stave off nausea, suddenly compelled by some inner voice to meet others who share his disease and its stigma, to lose himself in others that share his viral load, to acknowledge ontological difference but question the essentialism that might preclude a dissemination of the stories of HIVLTS. What right had I, a positive writer landing in Nairobi in 2009, *not* to seek out the stories of others growing older with the pandemic?[5]

Out in Africa

In 2009, a gay man in his fifties living in Montana, I was endeavouring, however half-heartedly, to wake every morning to count my blessings, thank gods, express gratitude for the light within, show amazement and delight that I was alive – I, who had been predicted to expire by the turn of the millennium, who contracted HIV in 1991 and now in 2009 was staying alive by ingesting daily protease inhibitors in Missoula. So why then did I dwell so regularly on the weeds in my garden, the come-ons from 20-something chubs, phone calls from relatives and friends who wanted money, letters, lessons, rides – everything and anything but a chance to talk to me about my life, to listen to my sadness, to ask about my upcoming trip to Africa, to Kenya for the poetry workshop?

By this time, the first African American president, whose father was Kenyan, had begun his $63 billion initiative on world health, a large portion of those funds destined for the United States President's Emergency Plan for AIDS Relief. Disgruntled as I was, I had much to be grateful for besides my survival. I was in the process of re-inventing myself as a poet; I was writing a novel; I was shopping a book of essays on queer film and the law. I had received a partial scholarship to study and write poetry at the

---

[5] Age is a relative term globally. In 2015, the life expectancy of an HIV-positive person living in sub-Saharan Africa was 54, and in some regions 49 (DoSomething.org, nd). A 20-year-old Ugandan on antiretroviral medication in 2011 had a 26.7-year life expectancy; in Canada and the United States, a man with HIV of the same age could expect 51.4 years (Wandeler et al, 2016).

Summer Literary Seminars in Nairobi.[6] Fancying myself as the next wannabe Longfellow, I was willing to cough up the extra thousand or two to get to Africa in December for a two-week workshop with Toi Derricotte, the magnanimous feminist African American who was short on discouraging words but fun to work with, even if I was a White male.

The flight to Kenya from Montana went through Amsterdam and took two days with the long layover. I carried my meds in a cool case in my daypack, concerned about lost luggage, nervous about customs and airport security. I might be pulled over in Kenya when immigration recognised the drugs; I might be turned back at the border for being a health risk. The flight from Amsterdam jammed me against a window looking out at darkness, at night, and climbing over unhappy geriatrics as I rose to urinate every 40 minutes, attempting to stay hydrated to avoid headaches that came anyway. I was still paying attention to raw egg and refusing lettuce in foreign lands. Tomato skins, crab cakes, raw tuna, the offer of Caesar salad – all verboten. I was also swallowing the requisite malaria medicine and dealing with its side effects.

I managed to arrive, in a grey van, at the rather elaborate pool and terraced hotel in the residential area of Nairobi the morning after. Earlier I had found the Summer Literary Seminars sign in the concourse of the Jomo Kenyatta International Airport and stepped into a crammed minivan. Looking at the other passengers, I wondered if I was the only *shoga* in the group, the only faggot. Was I the only one who, if by chance we crossed the border into Uganda, could be stoned to death if discovered kissing another man? I was surrounded by women from Boston and Brooklyn. I glanced about but only confirmed a feeling of isolation, ironically isomorphic with that on the Continental Divide from whence I had come. Travelling over poles, down to hemispheres made me no less anathema than I was as an out queer teacher in the Rocky Mountains.

Of course, water, sleep and pills were the orders of the day as I schlepped my luggage out of the clunking elevator and along to my fifth-floor room, where, door closed, I felt my hunger, felt the hammer on my cranium, felt the exhausted nervousness of my insular capsule of a room. Heading downstairs to the buffet, I eyed the sausages that swam in a sea of grease, my stomach almost erupting at the sight of pellucid corners of uncooked and tangled slabs of bacon. I found an empty table, powdered eggs, pale yellow segments jiggling with desiccation. I sat at a round table of nine chairs, half full. New arrivals spoke of contests and forthcoming novellas, dropping the names of keynote speakers. I had gained, with stiff nods of assent that seemed to resent my interruption of their brilliant repartee, permission to

---

[6] The Summer Literary Seminars involve two-week writing workshops in Canada, Kenya and Lithuania. The programme is affiliated with Concordia University in Montréal.

sit at their table, and sat in tongue-tied silence, sipping a tepid brew that slid down my throat with bowel-loosening ease. I had nothing to say for myself; I cringed at my awkward intrusion into the private convo of the literati, excused myself within minutes and headed back upstairs to my cubicle and the touch of a keyboard.

Kenya at 50

Asifuye mvuwa imemnyea [He who praises rain has been rained upon]

Kiswahili proverb

In the mirror there are no more imagos.
What I see are lines, furrows the sonnet warned about.
In these sockets, two blue fires stare out in fear.
At breakfast, no one asked about my dreams.
They glimpsed at crevices that once were cheeks.
Where would they have kissed me? Eyes averted to omelets,
among themselves they talked about giraffes, malaria.

I am at a conference in Kenya, staring at my face,
at the rough road from scalp to grizzle, the rift cratered,
lenses filmed with dust, crumbs. White coffee instant and weak.
I couldn't eat that tepid sausage, couldn't join their chat
    about photos,
couldn't feel these lips grow thinner in this simian jaw.
Shrunken. A pounding drum of jet lag behind my mask
told me to bite the stale pastry, spread the butter thick,

wipe my mouth and grin at dropped names. Bare a tooth, yellow
and long from gums that have receded. Did I ever belong?
Even when the squash players, splayed in the lounge, locked up
    my eyes,
even then, I knew their stare sterile. Even then coat sleeves
invited my veined and freckled arms. Five floors up I trudged,
eschewing strange and noisy elevators. I climbed to the top floor,
my heart burning. I turned the key and smelled my sleep.

In the mirror I see now what they would not look at.
    The graveyard,
strewn with bones. Pill tubes like fingers. Empty bottles
of plastic water, unabsorbed by skin. On the floor spines of tomes
unfinished. In the toilet, a ghost flushing three times.

He comes to bed with me. My friend, this jester, his fingers
at work through strands of my hair, his thumbs down my
   bent neck,
palms cupping my blurred vision. This rain, he says, will bless us.[7]

During our Kenya stay, we were introduced to members of Kwani, the local writers' organisation. During a Q and A after their round-table discussion, I had the postcolonial gumption to raise my hand and ask about the two Kenyan men who had recently married in London and were disowned by the country as a result. I asked them about the death Bill in neighbouring Uganda (ironically influenced by American evangelicals seeking to kill queers abroad if not allowed to do so at home). The question came at the end of the session and was answered with the kind of hurried discomfort that accompanies the appearance of elephants in living rooms, a metaphor that could in this context become literal on safari.

Sodomy is a felony in Kenya, requiring a 14-year sentence under Section 162 of the penal code, while 'gross indecency' (any sexual practice between men) carries a lesser 5-year sentence. Same-sex marriage is banned under the Constitution of Kenya, and the law has no explicit protections for sexual orientation or gender identity.[8] Kenya had one of the highest disapproval rating for homosexuality among 45 countries surveyed by the Pew Research Center in 2013, with 83 per cent of the polled populace finding homosexuality an unacceptable way of life. The Kenya Human Rights Commission (2011), which was recently allowed to do research in the country, found that 89 per cent of people who came out of the closet were disowned, ridiculed, assaulted, humiliated. Much of the opprobrium stems from the conservatism of Anglican bishops, Islamic sheiks and American evangelicals. Men who have sex with men are regularly assaulted by police or local militias, called *askaris*. Homosexuality, it goes without saying, is taboo in Kenya.

I jump ahead chronologically to share a few anecdotes that provide some context. In 2010, Prime Minister Odinga called it madness for a man to have sex with a man, since there are more women than men in Kenya. In the same year, close-caption cameras were installed in prisons to monitor

---

[7] 'Kenya at 50'first appeared in *Blood Work* (Charles, 2012) and *Zicatela* (Charles, 2018).

[8] The high court of Kenya upheld Sections 162 and 165 of the penal code on 24 May 2019, rebuffing a challenge by human rights organisations. Both laws were established under colonial rule in 1897, the first forbidding 'carnal knowledge against the order of nature' (14-year sentence) and the second banning 'indecent' acts between men (5-year sentence). In 2016 an appeals court ruled unconstitutional the law that allowed the police to conduct anal examinations on men arrested for same-sex behaviours (Equaldex, 2021).

contact. In 2011, the president of the Ksauni College put the blame for drought and inflation on people who engage in same-sex acts, while Obama, the tribal Kenyan, was warned by the Kenyan government to cease his gay-friendly speeches. In 2014, dozens of people were arrested in a Nairobi bar raid. Men who have sex with men (MSM)[9] are regularly blackmailed by police, evicted from homes and forced to move or close their businesses. In 2009, when two Kenyans, Charles Ngengi and Daniel Chege Gichia, became civil partners in a London ceremony, the event incited widespread condemnation throughout Kenya. Daniel's relatives were harassed in their village of Gathiru. In November 2017, when a photographer in the Maasai Mara captured an image of two male lions engaging in sexual mounting, Ezekiel Mutua of the Kenya Film Classification Board claimed that the animals had been 'influenced by gays who have gone to the national parks and behaved badly', leading to the animals' possession by 'demonic spirits' (Farrell, 2017).

The dangers surrounding anything queer in Kenya must have influenced even the left-wing literati of Kwani during their presentation at the seminar. The answers I received from the panellists about homosexuality were perfunctory, hushed and dismissive. Perhaps projecting, I felt politely frowned upon as an indiscreet American raising such a question, imposing his social and cultural 'values' through a colonialist presumptuousness. In my room, my friendly keyboard greeted me.

Shoga

The slang they use for men like me.
Kiswahili.
From the West, I bring this thing.
Un-African.
At the forum, I ask about their laws.
    Fourteen years for touch.
What about Uganda, the new death bill?
    Their neighbor nation.
What about those two men married in London,
    Kenyans cursed in Nairobi?
Bishops and hip hoppers united.
A kill-queer coalition.
They check their watches, cross their legs.
    No more time for questions.
I squirm in my chair, turn red,

---

[9] This is a term that avoids the labels of sexual identity, such as gay, straight or bisexual.

bite my pen.
They say, 'In Kenya, there are many phobias.
          Even dreadlocks.'
They say, 'We believe in democracy.
          Majority rule.'
What right have I to break taboo?
          Mzungu, foreigner.
How dare I raise my hand, a stone's throw from the slum?
          This silencer in me,
tourist from Montana, from a state blood red.
          Jaw breakers.
'Of course, it exists,' Billy tells me later. 'Late at night
          at clubs, you find them. At the Gypsy.
Go to big *hoteli*, go to the bar and drink.
Check websites for safaris.
In beach towns,' he whispers, 'it's more relaxed.'
          An undercurrent on the coast.

Though roseate and somewhat moist under arms after the conclusion of the panel discussion, I felt no regrets about asking these Kenyan intellectuals about the very oppression which international human rights and AIDS organisations were ascribing to the governments of East Africa. I felt proud of my audacity, proud of my concern for my fellow sodomites in a way that rather glaringly pointed out one of the prominent paradoxes that have informed the two great developments in my life. Of course, no one bothered to approach me in the courtyard after the session, but I was accustomed to being shunned. I could care less if they made the correct assumption that I was a *shoga*, a man who had sex with men, or even a *msenge*, a more formal term that suggested bottoming, for coming out had been the most momentous and courageous act of my life, an act that in fact had brought me the most joy and fulfilment sexually, emotionally, even to some degree socially.

For me, being queer was a delight even if a dangerous one – whether in Nairobi or Bozeman, Montana. It had nothing in the least to do with disease, mental or physical. But the irony of this embraced stigma became manifest in the other momentous event in my life, one that was in fact linked, however unfortunately, to the very struggle that had marked my romantic and even professional career, namely that being positive about being gay had led to HIV positivity, led in fact to the infection the mullahs and archbishops claim as proof of God's wrath on sick and unnatural perverts. The best thing that ever happened to me – my trip to the White Horse Bar in Oakland in 1980 – had somehow led to the most calamitous occurrence in my diary – the acquisition of a fatal virus. And no matter what silver lining I might ascribe to my long-term survival, no matter what lemonade from such a lemon – in terms of philosophy, meditation, poetry, intimations of mortality, even compassion – I would never be able to make peace with the cruel twist of fate that made my love lethal.

Coming out positive

Suffice it to say that I did not raise my hand at the colloquy and ask about the incidence of HIV in this sub-Saharan country, one of the worst affected in the world. I did not enquire about the stigmatisation of the 1.5 million people (almost 6 per cent of the population) living with the virus in 2010(Lupia and Chien, 2012). By 2014, Kenya shared fourth position, along with Mozambique and Uganda, in the list of countries with the highest per capita HIV populations – the high rate persists despite the decline in deaths and the increase in adults taking ARVs (Avert, 2020). Though women and children are hard hit in this country, new cases continue to find their primary hosts in key risk populations – men who have sex with men, drug users and sex workers. New cases are highest on the coast, and the prevalence of HIV is three times greater among my people than prominently heterosexual individuals – their incidence may be as high as one in five.

The good news is the widespread use of ARVs and the increase in testing as well as a fall from 100,000 to 62,000 new cases annually (Avert, 2020). PrEP is fully approved, and condom use is promoted, if more honoured in the breach rurally. Voluntary medical male circumcision – a controversial practice which nonetheless is said to lower conversion rates – is in full implementation. Also, the High Court of Kenya has held that mandatory disclosure of one's status is an unconstitutional infringement on individual rights – an anomalous but curiously important decision given the holier-than-thou attitude of Americans in the country who must live with the criminalisation of disclosure.[10]

The competing tensions of my identity, highlighted by this trip to a country where queer stigma was almost greater than that of HIV, led to some pressing curiosity during my first visit to East Africa. After the seminar, I stayed with friends in the suburbs south of Nairobi, in Karen, the area known as the Ngong Hills, made famous by Karen Blixen in her memoir *Out of Africa*. I reclined in the lap of luxury among the expats who hosted me. On making a requisite pilgrimage to Blixen's restored home, I recalled her early 20th-century stories of British colonialists in the 'happy hunting grounds', Kikuyi coffee farmers, roaming tribal Maasai hunters, migrating Somali Muslims and Indian merchants who came to Kenya to bank, lend, borrow and steal – but

---

[10] *SNW v. Asha Gulam Hat Case No. 003 of 2018*, Available from: http://kenyalaw.org/case law/cases/view/184441/

what pressed me as I sauntered across the cut lawns of Blixen's idyllic but eventually bankrupt farm, sold in the 1930s to Remy Martin, who subdivided it, was my strange and wistful nostalgia for my Thursday night HIV support group back home. I wondered what people like James and Randy were up to. Was there not a drop-in HIV spot, like an Alcoholics Anonymous meeting, where I might go to find queer positive Kenyans?

I suddenly felt compelled to find my people here, in one of the places deeply immersed in the travails of the AIDS struggle. Children, mothers, sex workers, truck drivers, closeted queers, MSM – all dying, all vying for ARVs. I had to find them, make some contact with them. They were probably were uninsured, probably far from the infectious disease specialist that insisted on a full examination of my lipoma-strewn body every six months. The ones who drew my blood, studied my lipid panels, my liver enzymes, my glucose levels, my triglycerides. The ones who listened to my heartbeat and drew wax from my contorted ear canals. What might it be like to be penniless, to live in Kibera, purportedly the largest slum in the world, to survive shunned and circumspect in the tight community of red dirt shacks with its maze of makeshift dwellings – what must it be like to live without all the modern conveniences, to live sometimes even without enough food, to wake up hungry and know too that you are viral, headed for sickness and suffering?

At first, I couldn't discern why I wanted desperately to connect with others who carried the burden of the HIV virus – why misery loves company – why I couldn't just enjoy myself with poets and writers and family and friends that peopled my little safari and beachcombing visit, scanning waves and hotel rooms for single men with whom I might make prolonged eye contact, if nothing else. The answer had its façade of altruism, its rehearsed intention of shedding light on the plight of others with the virus, of making the world aware of what we have experienced, as if detailing the lives of HIVLTS could somehow lead to a cure or social acceptance or boundary breaking. But this well-intentioned Mother Theresa cover had some darker sides, which I can now only fathom or plumb with trepidation, for to admit the self-promotion behind this project, behind any 'look at me and my problems' essay, requires a certain honesty that almost undermines the grander plan of narrating the lives of the untouchable and virtually quarantined queers with AIDS.

My enquiries about support groups arose out of some deep desire to commune, some longing to be with others like me – as if the witnessing or recognition of people who felt the burden of this microscopic and invisible load could lighten or help carry it. It was impossible even to understand what I was going through, let alone for me to understand the life of a single man in his thirties living in Kochi, one of the slums of Nairobi, living on what he could gain from part-time work – as if my awareness of his life could somehow make the hardship of that life, or mine, any less arduous. And yet the economy of communality, the value of revelation, the release that comes from unburdening one's soul among others with similar burdens cannot be measured by yardsticks of normal gain or loss. I may be availing myself of the mystery of the inexplicability of human contact as a way of rationalising my narrative, but to justify the ways of AIDS to men and women emerged as my life raft in this admittedly conflicted endeavour: to face the fact that I was gay and positive and that, yes, I was in the heart of HIV country and, yes, I better find out about it, to find myself in others – not as a way to somehow count my blessings, somehow underline the inequities of drug or medical supplies, not just to show how the other 90 per cent lives (though that was part of it), but something else. It was something about a confirmation in the eyes of others, about feeling what others feel – not as alleviation or some kumbaya moment of shared solidarity, but as a kind of witnessing, a kind of ciphering, an emptying out of what was left of the still detectable self in order to let the presence and timeline of others pour like rain, like a shower, through my body. There was a losing in listening, a loosening, a clearing out of the self through recognition of the trauma of others.

As a result of my persistence, I was dropped off at the offices of the Trust for Indigenous Culture and Health (TICAH) one morning.[11] The is an non-governmental organisation that promotes alternative health resources for underprivileged people in the slums. The women on salary – some from Kochi themselves – had been asked to accommodate the writer from Montana, to show him the offices and the mission of the organisation. I had not read through more than a couple of brochures before I asked point blank if there was an HIV support group I could attend while I was in town, and they, though decorous and I might say a little shocked, after some back-room confab, told me they would try to arrange a special meeting of the group in Kochi for Wednesday morning.

We drove by taxi from TICAH to the edge of the slum, a long drive north towards the city centre and then east to the township. From the car we could look out to the west at the vast uphill slope of Kibera. We were headed to Korogocho, however – another slum on the other side of the city. The driver stopped at a place where the intense iron orange road became too carved by erosive fissures to allow for motor vehicles. I walked with two other women, and as we moved up the road among skillets and goats and old men seated on crates, smoking, the sights and sounds of the thriving city within a city amazed me. A couple of times we moved off the wide main road into a maze of man-made alleys that led to dwellings, through a series of sharp, angular turns that left me easily lost in the warren. Alleyways were no wider than three feet, and living spots, almost all unpaved, were cordoned

---

[11] See https://www.ticahealth.org/np

off with corrugated plastic and old lumber. Some had roofs; few had floors. I was shaking hands with some smiling people and quickly shuffled off down the road to our eventual destination, a small room, maybe 80 square feet, where the couches and bed had been pushed against the wall and a bunch of chairs were set in a circle.

There were maybe six of us, maybe two guys (including me), the rest women. I introduced myself as a writer from the United States, a man who was living with HIV for over ten years. The walls of the room were covered with white sheets, and I was handed a cup of tea as we began to go around the circle, each person introducing herself to me, for I believe most everyone already was familiar with others in group. I remained in a daze as I listened to their stories and told my own. I did not mention my queerness, aware of the taboo.

Blood work

Come to the slum
Kochi, Nairobi
Scrap metal town
corrugated
dirt red.

My nonprofit guides
positive people
who peddle herbs and hope
take me through mazes
'how are yous' from kids
sweet homes built from junk.

This visitor
numb with privilege
shocked smiler
driven from his hotel
to see what he cannot feel.

We wend our way
through warrens
potholes
chickens in crates
charcoal cylinders.

To Mary's place
her door a dead car.

Inside, white sheets
cover walls
light the dark.

She burns incense
translates stories
from Swahili,
six in our group.
Ismael wants to find a lover
now the drugs have kicked in.

Saysa wants me to marry,
share her cabbage juice cocktail,
tell the world we are proud
to be alive with the virus.
She's made her body map
wears her *kanga* with a message.

Only Jedi quiets banter.
Below her lash
a tear appears.
She calls her brother Deus
the only one who did not shun her.

Her sniffle brings us close
close enough to close the circle.
It slides from duct to voice
speaks deeper than infection
sharper than stigma's sting
the way they stare at you like death
in Kochi, at home, in America.

Her tear immerses us
health workers, mothers
men who have sex
with men, writer intruder
who chokes on *asanti sanas*.

He took his pills this morning,
He rode the taxi to the center,
He wants to tell their story.
In silence they stand
chapped hands linked

like t-cells.
Blood work.

An intimate interview: Jane E

My encounter with the support group in Kochi inaugurated an extended project of collecting stories from long-term HIV survivors in different parts of the world. With free pens from my university and a handheld Toshiba recorder, I came back to Kenya in 2017 to listen to answers to a set of questions about conversion, tests, medications, disclosure, sexual relations before and after, about opportunistic infections, hospitalisations, doctors, expenses, about stigmas and taboos. In Kenya, my contacts were almost entirely with women, mostly ex-sex workers, in large part because of taboos around MSM activity and a reluctance of men to talk about HIV because of its common connection to sexual activity. I spent time in Nairobi's Majengo slum with my translator, recording the stories of long-term survivors living in a part of town known for sex work and HIV, but my home base was the TICAH office, housed in a set of one-storey brown-shingle cottages on a grand piece of land in the suburb of Nairobi called Karen. There are rose bushes and a gravel driveway. The setting is placid, befitting the cool climate of Kenya.

After I returned from a couple of interviews one morning, I stood around aimlessly until the office broke for lunch outside on picnic tables with some goat stew with rice laid out on a tablecloth. After lunch, Jane E, one of the staff of TICAH and my guide for the week, pulled up a chair beside me and told me she wanted to tell me her story. She spoke enough English that I didn't need a translator. She didn't want to be recorded, so I took some notes as we chatted about her life.[12]

Jane is from Homa Bay County near the section of Lake Victoria that borders southern Kenya. Somewhere near 40, today she wears a pink tufted and sparkled blouse, her hair pulled back, her heels high, her skirt a tight wrap-around. She has a smile as bright as a snowball and a laugh like a rough and happy hug. The village where she grew up and where she longs to return to after her TICAH work is done has a high incidence of HIV, she tells me, for two reasons: one cultural, the other economic (poverty). Men carry HIV and don't divulge it, and in her village if a brother dies, his brother has the option of marrying the widow. Marriage is often polygamous; men commonly spread the virus.

Jane is the eldest of 12 siblings. In August 1995, she followed her father, an askari (a security guard) to Nairobi. She was about 14, a virgin. One day

---

[12] I changed the names of the interviewee and her son in this account.

she accompanied a friend, who was about to marry, to get an HIV test at a nearby clinic. Back then, the test cost K Sh 500 (around €4), and Jane, who grew up in abject poverty and was now living in Kibera with her father, had no funds. On a lark, her friend said: "Get a test – why not, I'll pay for it." When Jane E came back two weeks later for the results, she sat in a large room in the clinic and her name was shouted out among a room full of people, including an older man who watched her closely. The doctor told her she had AIDS. He asked her where she got it. She said that she had no idea; she was a virgin, just in from the village; she was in school, her father scrounging up shillings for school fees. The doctor told her to leave. She got no counselling.

Jane figures she got the virus from a quack, a local medicine man in her village, when she was 12. She shows me the scar on her leg, where an abscess developed after a bad run-in with a stick when she was little. The "doc" stuck the swollen area with a needle that was probably quite unclean. Hence the virus, she tells me.

Back then, AIDS was a death sentence, so Jane decided to take the bull by the horns. She decided to kill herself before the disease killed her – slowly and painfully. Unfortunately, she ended up diluting the rat poison with water so thoroughly that she woke up after swallowing it to a world of vomit instead of an afterworld of HIV-less bliss. She refused to say anything to her solicitous father, who was quite worried about his firstborn daughter. Her second attempt came when she woke up at two in the morning, took a blanket and went to the railway line and curled up on the tracks to wait for the 4 o'clock train to end it all. A gang of three men found her and pulled her off the tracks, roughed her up and told her they were going to take her home. By some stroke of luck, they didn't rape her. Miffed, she led them to the wrong house, and they left her. She snuck back home after the guys took off.

Her dad wanted to know what in the name of heaven was going on, but Jane E kept her mouth shut, refusing to burden her father with her troubles. Thinking the third time the proverbial charm, she decided to try the highway south of Nairobi. She walked out into ongoing traffic and found herself resting on top of a car bonnet with no major injuries, the car more damaged than she was. A minor miracle basically. Jane was rushed to hospital and was released shortly thereafter. She finally decided that she was incapable of killing herself, so she gave up.

Jane left school, bitter and angry. Her father, in tears, asked her to tell him what the story was. She refused, she tells me, grinning with her big teeth, an infectious laugh exposing a dark spot on her upper gum. She left home at 15 and hung out in the slum with "the bad girls", getting into fights with her "friends" and the police, who dragged her home on occasion. She wasn't going to tell me if "hanging out" meant sex work.

One day, when the girls were fooling around at the Kenyatta market, a man came up to her and called her by name. "Jane," he said, "those girls are trouble." He told her not to be so bitter. He was older. He looked her in the eye and told her to calm down, to go back to her dad. "How the fuck did he know my name?" she wondered. Who was this guy, ten years older than she, becoming all paternalistic on her? The guy dragged her home to her dad and told her to meet him at the market the next day, but Jane E, rebellious and desperate, did not keep the appointment. She ignored her father's pleas for her to return to school. The mystery man returned to check up on her a few days later, and he offered to pay her school fees. He was just a tailor; he wasn't a rich man.

Jane eventually went back to school, and after a long courtship, she and tailor man became partners. She was 18. She gave birth to Samuel (her HIV-negative son and my translator in Majengo), but three years into their love, her man died of tuberculosis.[13] Jane was stuck with a baby and no job, forced to sell used clothes on the street. "Poor, poor, poor," she shakes her head. She can admit as much to me now, she says, now that she has married again (this time to a political worker), lives ten minutes from the posh suburb of Karen in a rented apartment, and has a nine-month-old child. Before, she wouldn't talk about that time to anyone.

After the death of Samuel's father, Jane E, who did not get on ARVs until last year, treated her condition herbally and decided to get involved as a counsellor for HIV children. Her interest in herbs led her to a talk at TICAH in 2008, where she met Mary Ann, the founder, and they became fast friends, bonding over alternative medicine. Jane started working hard to start support groups in the slums – Kochi, Kibera, Majengo, Kawangware. She did home healthcare for free; she became quite frenzied in her efforts to get people supported, tested, on herbs.

Jane decided to go back to Homa when she heard about the increasing incidence of AIDS deaths in her home town. A friend told her about the drug dumping pile in her village, a corner in the town where positives dumped their ARVs after receiving them free from the clinic. In Homa, clandestine, literally camped in the bushes for a day, Jane watched as four or five people came to the village pile and threw away their three-month supplies of nevirapine. Finally, she emerged and asked one woman what in the name of heaven she was doing. The drugs were making her sick, the emaciated women stated. The woman was malnourished and the drugs on an empty stomach were of course making her even sicker. Jane started

---

[13] Tuberculosis is a major cause of death in Kenya. In 2015, approximately 120,000 people contracted the disease (48,000 of them were HIV-positive), and it caused 18,600 deaths (Vassal, 2015).

crying; she couldn't believe it. The clinic was throwing generics at the population without even considering their socio-economic status or the fact they were starving.

Jane went to work with her usual zeal, organising support groups in her community, teaching about nutrition and herbs. She went door to door, convincing people to accept food, swallow herbs, stay healthy as they ingested the HIV meds they received. Eventually, after a couple of years, the support group she started swelled to 200 participants. She won a community award from The Egmont Trust in the United Kingdom and travelled there to make a presentation. After her talk, a donor came to her and offered to fund the support group. Later, some Japanese acquaintances offered to pay for building a clinic in her village. The pride of her life has been bringing deathbed patients back to life through support, dietary supplements and healthcare advice. Every weekend, she still travels back to her home town to hold group in her father's house, all her siblings now dispersed. A sudden gleam in her eyes attests to Jane's devotion to her village.

Once the excitement of detailing the Homa story settles down, Jane and I come back to our presence together under the shade of an acacia outside the TICAH office. I suddenly feel compelled to raise the issue of gender. I am an American man who, for the past week, has been interviewing carefully chosen middle-aged Kenyan women. Jane laughs about me joining the girls for lunch, a taboo that a foreign man can get away with since he knows no better. (Not until halfway through my goat stew did I notice the guys were eating separately over on a stone wall in the yard.) Don't worry, she tells me, some tribes do not even allow women to watch men eat. Jane, laughing, admits my interviews involve some knotty work. Women generally do not talk to men about sex, unless they are flirting.

When I bring up the question of MSM, Jane grows quieter, more circumspect. She knows guys are having sex, but it's a subject that never comes up. Same-sex relations are kept entirely under the table – entirely taboo (to use a culturally loaded term). People know guys are fucking and infecting one another, but most Kenyans refuse to acknowledge it. The church, colonial sodomy laws, prejudices over influences from the West – all have worked to make homosexuality un-African in the cultural imagination. So how can there be an awareness of HIV transmission if the behaviour that can spread it is itself anathema, unmentionable? In the world of Kenyan MSM practice, silence *does* equal death.

This leads to the larger problem of AIDS fatigue in Kenya, a country with one of the highest percentages of infected populations in the world. At that point in 2017, many Kenyans didn't want to talk about HIV any more. In 2002, the pandemic was so compelling that it was on the front burner by necessity. The media and the people had to take notice. People were dying. Now the slow puncture takes its time killing people, as those who get the drugs are managing it – those without, staying healthy for long as possible. The stigma of HIV has itself become silenced; people ignore it. Ironically, the pandemic has gone underground as treatments have improved. Now, AIDS is in the school textbooks, but it is still closeted in the community, except when someone finds your meds, at which point you are ostracised, slowly but surely. Sometimes the social consequences of being seen getting testing or taking the ARVs are so dramatic that people avoid the issue entirely, preferring to die.

Jane remains undaunted; she has dedicated her life to confronting HIV head-on. For now, she will continue as a TICAH worker, a support group organiser, an undetectable mother of two HIV-negative children. She's on the meds, happy living with her new husband. She's been to World AIDS Day events in Mexico, in Italy. She continues to speak on alternative medicine in her village, though the pharma people decry her claims about turmeric. Jane soldiers on – a survivor by example, an amazing star, making real change in her own Africa.

Because of the intimate nature of HIV in terms of its transmission and prognosis, many of my interviews with long-term survivors turned, suddenly, deeply emotional, for both me and the stranger I was questioning. Jane's story triggered amazement and admiration but also a kind of global sorrow and hope as I listened to the account of her life in Homa. Some scholars have compared interviewing to therapy, exploring the way the process of disclosure, especially around sexual issues, creates a space for confession, reflection and – in the process of conversation – a form of intercourse that in its own way partakes of a profound intimacy (Birch and Miller, 2000). The trauma of HIV – replete with its possibly fatal diagnosis, its dangerous remedies (like AZT), its alternative healing strategies (from faith to herbal remedies), its stigma and ostracism (sexual and social), its conspiracy theories, legal policing and pharmacological politics – asks the research participant to repeat, even relive, events that have combined Eros and Thanatos, the life and death drives, by means of a contagious and deadly virus contracted through the process of sexual pleasure.[14] What narrative could be more personal, more heart-wrenching, more difficult to divulge than the story of HIV – its contraction, its progress, its arrest, its suppression through costly drug regimens? In this way, both positive interviewer and positive interviewee re-enter and participate in a deeply disturbing re-experience of survival.

---

[14] Freud's *Beyond the Pleasure Principle*, published originally in 1920 (see Freud, 1961), is a speculative work that posits a struggle between Eros (the drive for sexual connection in part) and Thanatos (the death drive associated in part with self-destruction). What strikes me as deeply complex psychologically is the way experience of HIV, at least through sexual transmission, participates in both these conflicting drives.

When, at the end of her story, I asked Jane about MSM in Nairobi, I was also disclosing my own position as an older, gay, positive man confronting the struggles of endurance – socially, physically, emotionally – in a world that was at once entirely different from hers and, paradoxically, at the same time familiar. She wanted to know how long I had been positive, what drugs I was taking, who I was dating. She wanted to find out about me once I had found out about her. In this finding *out*, our worlds came together through a shared virus – global and virulent – that we both were striving to overcome.

References

Avert (2020) 'HIV and AIDS in Kenya' [online], Available from: https://www.avert.org/professionals/hiv-around-world/sub-saharan-africa/kenya np

Bersani, L. (1987) 'Is the rectum a grave?', *AIDS, Cultural Analysis/Cultural Activism*, 43: 197–227.

Birch, M. and Miller, T. (2000) 'Inviting intimacy: the interview as therapeutic opportunity', *International Journal of Social Research Methodology*, 3(3): 189–201.

Butler, J. (2004) *Precarious Life: The Powers of Mourning and Violence*, New York: Verso.

Charles, C. (2012) *Blood Work*, Lewisburg, PA: Seven Kitchens Press.

Charles, C. (2018) *Zicatela*, Kanona, NY: Foothills Publishing.

DoSomething.org (nd) 'Eleven facts about Africa' [online], Available from: https://www.dosomething.org/us/facts/11-facts-about-hiv-africa

Equaldex (2021) 'LGBT rights in Kenya' [online], Available from: https://www.equaldex.com/region/kenya

Farrell, J. (2017) 'Kenya official says male lions who had sex "must have seen gay men behaving badly" and should be separated', *Independent* [online], 3 November, Available from: https://www.independent.co.uk/news/world/africa/gay-lions-sex-kenya-photos-men-inspired-need-therapy-says-offic ial-a8036016.html

Fawcett, B. and Hearn, J. (2004) 'Researching others: epistemology, experience, standpoints and participation', *Social Research Methodology*, 7(3): 201–18.

Freud, S. (1961) *Beyond the Pleasure Principle: The Standard Edition*, trans J. Strachey, New York: Liveright.

Jackson, J.B. (2021) 'On cultural appropriation', *Journal of Folklore Research*, 58(1): 77–122.

Johnston, A. (2018) 'Jacques Lacan', in E.N. Zalta (ed) *Stanford Encyclopedia of Philosophy* [online], Available from: http://plato.cstandord.edu/archives/fall2018/entries/lacan/

Kenyan Human Rights Commission (2011) *The Outlawed Amongst Us: A Study of the LGBTI Community's Search for Equality and Non-Discrimination in Kenya* [online] Available from: https://www.khrc.or.ke/mobile-publi cations/equality-and-anti-discrimination/70-the-outlawed-amongst-us/ file.html

Lupia, R. and Chien, S.-C. (2012) 'HIV and AIDS epidemic in Kenya: an overview', *Journal of Experimental and Clinical Medicine*, 4(4): 231–4.

UNAIDS (nd) 'Global HIV & AIDS statistics—fact sheet' [online], Available from: https://www.unaids.org/en/resources/fact-sheet

Vassal, A. (2015) 'Kenya perspective: tuberculosis', *Copenhagen Consensus Center* [online], Available from: https://www.copenhagenconsensus.com/ publication/kenya-perspective-tuberculosis

Wandeler, G., Johnson, L.F and Egger, M. (2016) 'Trends in life expectancy of HIV-positive adults on ART across the globe: comparisons with general population', *Current Opinion in HIV AIDS*, 11(5): 492–500.

9

Survival of an older Bangladeshi lesbian experiencing intersectional vulnerability

Kanamik Kani Khan

Introduction

Living as an older gender or sexually diverse person in a society that stigmatises and oppresses gender and sexually diverse communities is challenging. Many gender and sexually diverse people in Bangladesh live by hiding their identities to avoid social stigma and exclusion. The patriarchy and male-dominant values play a significant role in the experiences of gender and sexually diverse populations, especially lesbians. This chapter focuses on the case of an older lesbian, referred to here as Didi. Older people are disadvantaged in many parts of the world due to inadequate financial support and lack of health provisions and social care (Kneale et al, 2021). Didi's experience of what it is like to live as an older lesbian is used here as a lens to tell us what it is like to live a diverse identity while also needing to get access to health and social care and having social relationships. This chapter also investigates the role of religion in Didi's life as well as implications for mental health, resilience and support for people living with HIV, based on her lived experiences.

Didi's experience gives us insight into how stigma can be intersectional for an older woman who also identifies as a lesbian in postcolonial Bangladesh. The stigma older lesbians experience in Bangladesh sits at the intersection of oppression by men, prejudice related to sexual diversity and ageism. While there are challenges in using one person's experience to explore issues for wider populations, Didi's experience – due to the nature of her work – is a useful lens. This chapter conveys her multifarious insights about living at the intersection of multiple stigmas and how this impacts her mental health. Didi's experience in providing support for people living with HIV is discussed in order to reflect how the government regulates health provision for people living with HIV.

Background

This chapter is based on findings from doctoral research that investigated healthcare experiences of gender and sexually diverse communities in

Bangladesh. A phenomenological approach was taken to examine the lived experiences of the participant in order to understand what it is like to be a gender or sexually diverse person, an ageing person or a person living with HIV in a society that is culturally conservative. I used qualitative methods, particularly in-depth interviewing, and thirteen participants were recruited for the study. Since gender and sexually diverse people are mostly hidden and considered as 'hard to reach' populations in Bangladesh, to get closer to this group, I worked as a volunteer with a local agency that works (not publicly) with gender and sexually diverse communities. Through this volunteer role, I was able to build trust and networks, and interact with gender and sexually diverse people in person to better understand their world views regarding life, sexuality and religion. This role also allowed me to recruit study participants. I chose to present Didi's story in this chapter as a way of reflecting the local context and understanding the complex nature of oppression in Bangladesh.

Didi's story

Didi lives in urban Bangladesh and is in her early sixties. She had her 'self-identification' when she was about 11 years old. The notion of self-identification is equivalent to the Western concept of 'coming out', or disclosing one's variant sexual or gender identity to oneself and others. This was a very important moment in Didi's life; self-identification was a difficult journey for her, as she did not have any understanding of the concepts of same-sex relationships or sexual and gender diversity. She is Muslim and holds her faith in Islam, and she expressed that every religion emphasises support for marginalised people. Didi is an educated person and very career oriented; she has worked in different occupations. Currently, she works for Bijito (a pseudonym for an organisation that works with gender and sexually diverse communities in Bangladesh) as a focal person – a person authorised by an organisation to represent members – to support young gender and sexually diverse people, including those living with HIV, through counselling, awareness-building and emotional support. She believes education should be the utmost priority in life because, regardless of what society one lives in or one's sexual or gender diversity, education can always help a person to fight injustice, oppression and marginalisation.

Sexuality is regarded as a very private matter and is often a taboo in Bangladesh (Riaz and Rahman, 2016), so there is little public discussion or awareness about gender and sexuality. This is one of the reasons Didi was inspired to work with an organisation that helps to build social awareness about nonconforming genders and identities. Didi stressed the value of education:

'Educating each unit of society [family] can be a way to bring change and build social awareness gradually. For this, I provide counselling to family members or parents of young gender and sexually diverse people to help them understand more about gender and sexually diverse identities.'[1]

However, she described that it is difficult to educate society as a whole, especially when voicing issues about same-sex relationships can be a threat to life. Two gay activists, Xulhaz Mannan and Mahbub Rabbi, in Bangladesh were assassinated by extremists in 2016. Ansar al-Islam (the Bangladeshi division of al-Qaeda) claimed responsibility for the killings, despite the claim of the Home Minister that there were no branches of Islamic State or al-Qaeda in Bangladesh (Sanzum, 2017).

Didi as a lesbian in a patriarchal society

Bangladesh is a South Asian nation that from 1947 to 1971 was known as East Pakistan. Before that, it was a part of India, which was ruled as a colony by the British for almost 200 years. Due to this history, Bangladeshi culture is influenced by many colonial values. Stoler (1989, as cited in Benard, 2016), a feminist scholar, introduces the concept of 'who could bed and who could wed' as one of the fundamentals in the construction of the British colony. This concept refers to the colonial assumption that women of colour can only be involved in prostitution and concubinage, and that only White women could be married and share the status of her husband. This exposes women of colour to sexual exploitation (Benard, 2016). Such racialised colonial gender norms were imported into the South Asian regions. *Sati*, a Hindu ritual in which a widow immolates herself on her husband's funeral pyre, and several Islamic religious interpretations further contribute to maintaining patriarchal dominance and continuing the oppression of gender identities outside the norm. Consequently, nonconforming genders are regarded as socially deviant and marginalised (Bondyopadhyay and Ahmed, 2011).

The rights of women have been traditionally suppressed in Bangladesh through the use of religious interpretations and conservative values (Cain et al, 1979). In 1972, following Bangladesh becoming independent in 1971, the country's constitution established women's rights as equal to those of men; all citizens, irrespective of gender, are equal before the law and entitled to have equal protection under the law (Momen et al, 1995; Ameen, 2005). In addition to the constitution, other national policies and guidelines emphasise the protection of women's rights. Even so, in many cases, women are not

---

[1] Quotes have been translated from Bengali by the author.

allowed to participate in the decision-making process in socio-economic, familial and political matters (Banarjee, 2020). Moreover, women have only limited rights or access in such areas as rights to education, health, social security, nutrition, shelter and freedom of expression (Chowdhury, 2003; Ameen, 2005).

Gender has also had a significant impact on property inheritance (Abdullah et al, 2014). Although equal rights for men and women is emphasised in many Western discourses (Khan et al, 2016), equal property distribution is not considered fair from an Islamic perspective (Barlow and Akbarzadeh, 2006). Women are legally deprived of their right to property in Islamic jurisdictions, with a son getting double what a daughter inherits, following the Quran, 4:11 (Khan et al, 2016). Despite this, the Bangladeshi government – based on its National Women's Development Policy (2011), which aims to ensure equal rights and opportunities for women (Tusher, 2011) – legislated for equal rights to property and inheritance for women and men. This amendment was protested by many religious communities though it was argued to be a political matter (Khan et al, 2016). But the protest was justified as an expression of patrinormativity (a concept that regards male-dominant values as the default) by cis-het men insisting on using religion to serve the purpose of maintaining male dominance. Therefore, although in theory women and men are equal, in practice religious theology has replaced government policy to maintain cisgender heterosexual male dominance, with religious interpretations being used to deprive women of their rights (Cain et al, 1979). Moreover, cis-het men work to ensure that it is not only women who are subordinated, but anyone who threatens to destabilise existing social norms, structures and privileges. Hence, all gender and sexually diverse people are similarly affected by the use of religion. They are denied equality and have no constitutional or other legal protections.

Although Didi grew up in a predominantly patriarchal society (Karim et al, 2018), she was raised in an educated family with very little prejudice. As a result, she was able to continue her education, even though female education was not a common practice in most Bangladeshi families during the 1970s (Raynor, 2005). Although she was in love with a woman, as a result of social and family pressures she married a man; she is now divorced. Marriage is a social expectation in Bangladesh, and every family directly or indirectly puts pressure on their children to get married. Didi reported that because of patriarchy, lesbians are in a situation where they are unable to protest forced marriage, although in many cases, gay men can do so. Didi said: "Like me, many gender and sexually diverse individuals are forced to get married without their consent, because same-sex relationships are not socially accepted."

This kind of forced marriage is common due to Section 377 of the Indian Penal Code (1860). This criminalises homosexual behaviour and regards same-sex relationships as 'unnatural'. Thus, many gender and sexually diverse individuals are left with no other choice but to participate in forced marriages. Section 377 was introduced under British rule and is still a part of the law in Bangladesh. Religious norms and patriarchal values about gender and sexuality – mostly derived from the British colonial era – contribute to the expectation of gender conformity in Bangladeshi society, where most people deem same-sex relationships to be deviant (Ferdoush, 2013).

Impact of religion

Gender and sexually diverse individuals from a Judaeo-Christian background often find that their religion and their identities conflict (Guittar, 2013; Hamblin and Gross, 2014). In fact, in many cases, gender and sexually diverse people consider religion to be more of a hindrance than a support in their lives (Henrickson, 2007). In one study, gender and sexually diverse people with high religious affiliation were more likely than heterosexual people with similar views to have suicidal thoughts and even to attempt self-harm (Lytle et al, 2018). However, limited studies have been conducted on this conflict within Muslim populations. Gany and Subhi (2018) point out that those that have been conducted tend to be in countries with a Muslim minority (such as Bangladesh, India, Iran, Iraq and Pakistan). Didi explained that she holds her faith in Islam strongly; however, she said: "Due to the nature of my work, I interact with many gender and sexually diverse people who think that religion is a barrier to identifying and disclosing themselves to others."

Didi observed that while religious attitudes deem sex and sexuality for pleasure to be bad, sex for reproduction is viewed as necessary. She noted that sexual practices which do not lead to reproduction (such as fornication, pornography, same-sex practices, masturbation and artificial contraception) are regarded as sinful in Roman Catholic theology (The Holy See, nd). Similarly, the view of Orthodox Judaism implies that homosexual behaviour should be prohibited (Lamm, 1974). Islamic understandings are similar. For instance, Islamic scholars, including the popular Egyptian cleric Yusuf al-Qaradawi, argue that there is no restriction on oral sex between husband and wife as long as no semen is released; if this happens then the oral sex is *makruh* (blameworthy). Yusuf's view is very popular because there is no clear command or evidence in the Hadith or the Quran prohibiting this act (Keating, 2012). On the other hand, a common censure against Yusuf's view is that mouth and tongue are used for recitation of the Quran and the remembrance of Allah, hence oral sex should not be performed (al-Hudha, 2001). The main argument comes down to whether sex is for pleasure or reproduction. Didi believed that this conflict is one of the many modalities of a patriarchal society that forces gender and sexually diverse people, whose sexual expression is not for reproduction, to experience social rejection due to their religion.

Didi as an older lesbian

Although Didi does not have any major health problems, she mentioned that as a person ages, they can experience different kinds of health issues. Both physical and mental health issues are common in older Bangladeshis. Some common types of physical health problems experienced by the older population in Bangladesh are dementia, fatigue, hearing and vision problems, asthma, high blood pressure and chest pain. Loneliness as a result of social isolation is another issue experienced by this group (Kabir et al, 2013). Didi stressed that mental health issues are severe among older gender and sexually diverse communities. She explained that since she does not usually disclose her sexual orientation when visiting a healthcare setting, she is unlikely to experience any adverse reaction from the healthcare professionals. However, she thought that such as disclosure can become an extra burden alongside one's condition, because it can lead to stigmatising and discriminating healthcare experiences that can exacerbate the existing health problems. This can be more of an issue at an older age, as one's health is more likely to worsen.

Didi explained that lesbians often suffer from urinary tract infections as they sometimes fail to maintain personal hygiene, and they rarely disclose the infection to physicians. She also said that such infections can lead to depression. For lesbians, the fear of the discovery of their sexuality also affects routine healthcare consultations. For example, if a lesbian cannot express her sexuality or explain her sexual behaviours properly, the physician may not be able to advise her on how to maintain good hygiene. Didi said:

> 'Many people who call us on the helpline want to know how to have safe sex, and we explain it to them. We explain to them how to maintain hygiene in this situation. Those who are in my network suffer relatively less from this problem, but those who are not in my network may suffer terribly from such problems and cannot even go to the doctor.'

Didi said that while many healthcare professionals believe healthcare is a fundamental for everyone, they are often reluctant to put this into practice when it comes to interacting and providing medical treatment to gender and sexually diverse people. This is one reason why many older gender and sexually diverse people do not feel able to disclose their identity in a healthcare setting.

Didi explained that social care is not sufficiently considered in Bangladesh. Research suggests that the rising share of the population who are aged over

70 years will lead to an increasing care deficit (Kabir et al, 2013). Agencies (for example, care homes) and government institutions that provide care for older people do not have adequate resources to provide care for the increasing number of older persons. According to Didi, this is because the cost of long-term care for older persons is simply too high for a developing country. Didi further explained that there is a social stigma about care homes for older persons in Bangladesh, a society where people tend to believe that sending an elder family member to a care home is avoidance of parental responsibility. Avoiding this responsibility is taboo in Bangladeshi culture, as people are culturally bound to live together with their family members of all generations. This is particularly a problem for gender and sexually diverse older people who no longer have ties with their blood kin, so do not have families of their own to care for them. The stigma of residential care for older people must be removed in order to provide for the needs of older people effectively (Iraj, 2019). Didi described that when older people are seen as a burden, whether to family, society or state, they are already in a position of disadvantage and stigmatised; living as a gender and sexually diverse person multiplies the experience of stigma.

Didi recounted a meeting with government officials where she frequently used the term 'transgender' and insisted on the relevance of sexuality and gender in planning. Throughout, a government official whispered to her that she should use the term 'hijra' instead of 'transgender', as the latter brought concepts of sexuality and gender diversity into the discussion, which was discouraged in that context. Hijra are individuals who have birth sex of male but present themselves and live as females, or as neither male nor female (Hinchy, 2019). Sometimes, transgender and intersex persons are also identified as hijra in Bangladesh. This episode is an example of government officials not accepting the public discussion of sexuality and people with different sexual and gender characteristics. As a result, the concepts and interventions for sexual health and the other health needs of these communities remain underdeveloped. Didi said:

'The government is reluctant to discuss sexuality and they believe that there are no [gender and sexual minority] populations in Bangladesh. Despite knowing about sexuality and gender interrelated concepts, they never acknowledge it. So how can we expect support from the Government when they do not believe we exist?'

Older people can be somewhat dependent on others, and the level of dependency tends to increase with age (Islam and Nath, 2012). Extra financial support may be required. In Bangladesh, under the Old Age Allowance in the financial year 2021–22, each beneficiary received Tk 500 (US$5.83) per month (Department of Social Services, 2021). Didi compared this to the average monthly income in Bangladesh, which was an estimated Tk 13,258 (US$154.58) in 2017 (Trading Economics, 2021), arguing that the amount of money provided by the allowance was not enough to survive on. Furthermore, while COVID-19 has financially affected almost all people and business enterprises in Bangladesh, older persons are among the worst affected (Help Age International, 2020). For Didi, with this level of economic vulnerability, older people are already overlooked by the state, and being an older lesbian adds an extra layer of vulnerability due to the stigma towards gender and sexually diverse populations.

Support for people living with HIV

HIV first appeared in Bangladesh in 1989, and because of robust outreach and prevention efforts, it remains a relatively low-incidence country. According to Health and Family Welfare Minister Zahid Malik, a total of 7,374 individuals were living with HIV in Bangladesh in 2019; however, the actual number of people living with HIV is estimated at roughly 14,000 (Amin, 2019). This is arguably not an alarming number given the size of the population (163 million in 2019[2]). The United Nations International Children's Emergency Fund (UNICEF, nd) reports that HIV affects only 0.1 per cent of the overall population, although recent data indicate that new cases of infection are increasing. The wide range of estimates of people living with HIV reflects the lack of testing, either because testing is unavailable or because people are unwilling to go for tests. Two thirds of the HIV cases are returning migrant workers and their spouses (Urmi et al, 2015); injection drug users (IDUs) also constitute a relatively large group of people with HIV, and in one study HIV prevalence among street-based IDUs was found to be 7 per cent (Reddy et al, 2008). Sex workers also constitute a group at significant risk (Paul, 2019). The data on HIV suggest that HIV infections are more prevalent among migrant workers and IDUs than in gender and sexually diverse communities. Thus, one could argue that the initial focus of international aid on gender and sexually diverse communities averted a more serious outbreak in the latter. However, Didi expressed concern that if foreign donations and funds decrease and national government priorities come into force, the number of HIV infections may rise.

HIV testing and counselling (HTC) units or centres provide both voluntary and provider-initiated testing and counselling (Kennedy et al, 2013). The International Centre for Diarrhoeal Research Bangladesh established the first HTC unit in 2002, and more units were created with support from various non-governmental organisations (Urmi et al, 2015). However,

---

[2] Source: https://www.worldometers.info/world-population/bangladesh-population/

access to HTC is still insufficient in Bangladesh due to the limited numbers of units as well as stigma against people living with HIV (National AIDS/STD Programme, 2016).

HIV-related services have become more limited in recent years, one reason being the reduction in foreign donations for HIV prevention. Didi said:

'Donations have decreased, the projects or funding that we used to get in the past for HIV prevention are no longer available. There were two projects operated by The Global Fund but now there is only one Global Fund project for HIV prevention. Our healthcare services started to be limited as the project shut down or the funds decreased.'

Another reason for reduction of HTC units and HIV services is that services are gradually being shifted to government hospitals. Didi said:

'The government has moved many HTC units from NGOs to government hospitals, and this has created a concern for disclosure. One disadvantage of relocating many HTC units into government hospitals is that visiting a government hospital for HIV testing can increase the risk of public humiliation and insult to gender and sexually diverse populations.'

It is worth noting that the role of HTC is to prevent HIV, and many gender and sexually diverse people visit HTC units for prevention services. Not all gay men engage in anal intercourse, but this is a common route of HIV transmission for men who have sex with men (Grov et al, 2015). Didi explained that even though anal intercourse is just one of the ways HIV is transmitted, the general public is unwilling to believe that there are other transmission routes; thus, the stigma towards gender and sexually diverse populations is also expressed towards people living with HIV.

It is possible that the government has been gradually and quietly absorbing HTC units so as not to attract the attention of the media or the public. Didi expressed concern that the government is perhaps trying to maintain social control and oppression over these groups by requiring them to go to government hospitals for HIV testing and services. Didi further explained that HIV testing in government hospitals perceived as more dangerous for gender and sexually diverse people, because they do not know how healthcare providers and other staff will react to them. HIV testing in NGOs was viewed more positively, as most non-governmental organisation staff tend to be relatively supportive of gender and sexually diverse communities. Thus the relocation of many HTC units from NGOs to government hospitals may create a sense of fear among gender and sexually diverse people, which in turn affects their overall health-seeking behaviour.

Didi stated that the number of HIV-infected people increases every year and that this should be a concern for government. She said that the government cannot just disregard this fact and say that HIV is not a big health issue because of its apparent lack of consequences on public health. Didi stated:

> 'About one hundred Rohingya [refugees from Myanmar] individuals have been detected with HIV; many agencies are worried that the number of HIV infections per annum may increase further. Therefore, HIV has remained a big concern for public health and there is no point in taking HIV for granted.'

Didi's mental health and resilience as an older lesbian

As an older lesbian, Didi had suffered from depression, and she required medical attention for this. She was prescribed different kinds of powerful antidepressant medicines that negatively affected her health. Consequently, her work life was affected as she simply could not attend work. Due to frequent absences, she received a notice about how she is doing or whether she wanted to continue to work. Didi stated:

> 'The notice was an indirect message that they do not want me to return to work any more. The medicines were too powerful [and] made me sleep most of the time ... and I felt dizziness during the time I was awake. I knew I could not go on like this and I needed to change my attitude of feeling like a failure.'

After two weeks of suffering like this, she stopped taking the medications and left her job, where she had been unhappy. She immediately went to the office of the organisation where she is currently employed and asked to work to support gender and sexually diverse people in any way she could. With her previous work and life experience, the organisation was happy to employ her. Didi explained that lack of awareness among the general public about mental health issues is one factor that pushed her to switch careers. She thought if mental health support was not provided for people in need, gender and sexually diverse minorities are unlikely to have their well-being addressed.

Although Didi had to quit her previous job, her experience with depression as an older lesbian made her more aware of how to manage depression and build resilience among older people. She explained that an older person needs to appreciate something already present and good in their life; she referred to this as "practising gratitude". The feeling of gratitude activates the regions of the human brain that are concerned with the neurotransmitter dopamine; dopamine usually makes a person feel good thus it is regarded as a reward neurotransmitter (Olguín et al, 2016). Also, dopamine encourages the initiation of action, so an increased level of dopamine can make a person do something good again and again (Ko and Wanat, 2016). Ng et al (2012), in their study of the combined impacts of gratitude and sleep quality on anxiety and depression, found that a person with a higher degree of gratitude sleeps better, and people who practise gratitude are less likely to be depressed. Didi said: "An older gender and sexually diverse person can go through depression due to the stigma and vulnerability he/she experiences due to being an older and a marginalised person. Therefore, having some awareness about how to manage depression is very important to develop emotional wellbeing and mental health."

Older gender and sexually diverse people who live or stay connected with their communities tend to receive social support and grow their sense of belonging (Fredriksen-Goldsen, 2014). This could be one of the reasons why Didi made the decision quite consciously to change her career and to work with gender and sexually diverse communities – to develop the sense of belonging that contributes to her resilience. Didi runs training and awareness-building workshops with gender and sexually diverse communities. She did not see these as leisure activities, but rather as activities that result in a substantially higher degree of positive health and a better quality of life (Fredriksen-Goldsen, 2014).

Another factor that may have contributed to her resilience is her love life. Didi fell in love with a woman at a young age; they mostly spent time together at home and the family did not suspect anything since they were both girls. Williams and Fredriksen-Goldsen (2014) state that for older gender and sexually diverse people, maintaining same-sex relationships is associated with more positive mental health and fewer depressive symptoms compared with older gender and sexually diverse people who are single. Didi said: "Some friends noticed our relationship and they were generally supportive. Back then, although we were together, we did not have any understanding of the concepts of same-sex relationships or the concept of gender and sexually diverse identities." But their love was not socially accepted, and due to social pressure, Didi's female partner had to get married to a man; this resulted in Didi's depression at a very young age. Later, Didi also had to marry a man. But after her divorce, she and her ex-female partner got back in touch. Didi did not say explicitly that they were back together again, because her ex-partner is still married to a man. Notwithstanding, Didi felt that reuniting after a long time with the person she has been in love with for many years was an important contributor to her resilience.

Conclusion

Didi's lived experience and willingness to share her story allow us to understand something about what it is like to live as an older lesbian in a male-dominant society. Her personal and social life, her access to health and social care, her career have all been significantly affected by the predominant patriarchal values. Her struggles as an older lesbian suggest that it is not easy to live as a lesbian or as a person with HIV in Bangladesh, especially as society and the majority of the population continue to oppress women or accept the oppression of women as the way things are. Additionally, the economic vulnerability and stigma faced by older people can intensify the struggles of an older lesbian. Her lived experience of depression and recovery from it tells us a unique journey of reviving mental health. Didi's viewpoint and her learnings and observations from working with gender and sexually diverse communities allow us to understand how religion can impact gender and sexually diverse communities' understandings of self, access to health and social care, and engagement in relationships. Didi's experiences of intersectional oppression and observations as an older lesbian provide a lens that allows insight into what it is like to live an identity that sits outside enforced cultural norms.

References

Abdullah, R., Radzi, W.M., Johari, F. and Dastagir, G. (2014) 'The Islamic legal provisions for women's share in the inheritance system: a reflection on Malaysian Society', *Asian Women*, 30(1): 29–52.

al-Hudha, A.A. (2001) 'Remembrance of Allaah', Islamic Network [online], Available from: https://web.archive.org/web/20120415032643/http://www.islaam.net/main/display.php?id=391&category=134

Ameen, N. (2005) *Wife Abuse in Bangladesh: An Unrecognised Offence*, Dhaka, Bangladesh: The University Press.

Amin, M.A. (2019) '919 HIV infected, 170 die from AIDS in 2019', *Dhaka Tribune* [online], 1 December, Available from: https://www.dhakatribune.com/bangladesh/2019/12/01/919-hiv-infec ted-170-dies-from-aids-in-2019

Banarjee, S. (2020) 'Identifying factors of sexual violence against women and protection of their rights in Bangladesh', *Aggression and Violent Behavior* [online], 52: 101384. doi: 10.1016/j.avb.2020.101384

Barlow, R. and Akbarzadeh, S. (2006) 'Women's rights in the Muslim world: reform or reconstruction', *Third World Quarterly*, 27(8): 1481–94.

Benard, A.A.F. (2016) 'Colonizing Black female bodies within patriarchal capitalism: feminist and human rights perspectives', *Sexualization, Media, & Society* [online], 2(4). doi: 10.1177/2374623816680622

Bondyopadhyay, A. and Ahmed, S. (2011) *Same-Sex Love in a Difficult Climate: A Study into the Life Situation of Sexual Minority (Lesbian, Gay, Bisexual, Kothi and Transgender) Persons in Bangladesh*, Dhaka, Bangladesh: Bandhu Social Welfare Society.

Cain, M., Khanam, S.R. and Nahar, S. (1979) 'Class, patriarchy, and women's work in Bangladesh', *Population and Development Review*, 5(3): 405–38.

Chowdhury, A. (2003) *Violence against Girls in Bangladesh*, Dhaka, Bangladesh: Bangladesh Institute for Human Rights.

Department of Social Services (2021) 'Old Age Allowance', *Department of Social Services, Government of the People's Republic of Bangladesh* [online], 24 August, Available from: http://www.dss.gov.bd/site/page/7314930b-3f4b-4f90-9605-886c36ff423a/Old-Age-Allowance

Ferdoush, M.A. (2013) 'Living with stigma and managing sexual identity: a case study on the kotis in Dhaka', *Sociology Mind*, 3(4): 257–63.

Fredriksen-Goldsen, K.I. (2014) 'Despite disparities, most LGBT elders are aging well', *Aging Today* [online], 35(3), Available from: https://www.ncbi.nlm.nih.gov/pmc/articles/PMC4243168/

Gany, M.Y.D. and Subhi, N. (2018) 'Religious and sexual identity conflict among same-sex attracted Muslim men: a conceptual differences of life experience between Western and Muslim majority countries', *Jurnal Psikologi Malaysia,* 32(4): 133–49.

Grov, C., Rendina, H J., Moody, R.L., Ventuncac, A. and Parsons, J.T. (2015) 'HIV serosorting, status disclosure, and strategic positioning among highly sexually active gay and bisexual men', *AIDS Patient Care and STDs*, 29(10): 559–68.

Guittar, N.A. (2013) 'The meaning of coming out: from self-affirmation to full disclosure', *Qualitative Sociology Review*, 9(3): 168–87.

Hamblin, R.J. and Gross, A.M. (2014) 'Religious faith, homosexuality, and psychological well-being: a theoretical and empirical review', *Journal of Gay & Lesbian Mental Health*, 18(1): 67–82.

Help Age International (2020) *Income Security for all Older People in Bangladesh during COVID-19 and Beyond*, Dhaka, Bangladesh: Help Age International, Available from: https://www.helpage.org/silo/files/income-security-for-all-older-people-in-bangladesh-during-covid19-and-beyond.pdf

Henrickson, M. (2007) 'Lavender faith: religion, spirituality and identity in lesbian, gay and bisexual New Zealanders', *Journal of Religion & Spirituality in Social Work: Social Thought*, 26(3): 63–80.

Hinchy, J. (2019) *Governing Gender and Sexuality in Colonial India: The Hijra, c. 1850–1900*, Cambridge: Cambridge University Press.

The Holy See (nd) 'Catechism of the Catholic Church – Part three: life in Christ' [online], Available from: https://www.vatican.va/archive/ENG0015/__P5D.HTM

Iraj, S. (2019) 'Old age homes: remove the stigma', *The Independent* [online], 9 November, Available from: https://theindependentbd.com/post/223035

Islam, M.N. and Nath, D.C. (2012) 'A future journey to the elderly support in Bangladesh', *Journal of Anthropology*: 752521. doi: 10.1155/2012/752521

Kabir, R., Khan, H.T., Kabir, M. and Rahman, M.T. (2013) 'Population ageing in Bangladesh and its implication on health care', *European Scientific Journal*, 9(33): 34–47.

Karim, R., Lindberg, L., Wamala, S. and Emmelin, M. (2018) 'Men's perceptions of women's participation in development initiatives in rural Bangladesh', *American Journal of Men's Health*, 12(2): 398–410.

Keating, J.E. (2012) 'Sex and the single mullah', *Foreign Policy* [online], 23 April, Available from: https://foreignpolicy.com/2012/04/23/sex-and-the-single-mullah/

Kennedy, C.E., Fonner, V.A., Sweat, M.D., Okero, F.A., Baggaley, R. and O'Reilly, K.R. (2013) 'Provider-initiated HIV testing and counseling in low and middle-income countries: a systematic review', *AIDS and Behavior*, 17(5): 1571–90.

Khan, I., Abdullah, M.F. Rahman, N.N.A., Nor, M.R.B.M. and Yusoff, M.Y.Z.B.M. (2016) 'The right of women in property sharing in Bangladesh: can the Islamic inheritance system eliminate discrimination?', *SpringerPlus* [online], 5(1): 1695. doi: 10.1186/s40064-016-3347-2

Kneale, D., Henley, J., Thomas, J. and French, R. (2021) 'Inequalities in older LGBT people's health and care needs in the United Kingdom: a systematic scoping review', *Ageing & Society*, 41(3): 493–515.

Ko, D. and Wanat, M.J. (2016) 'Phasic dopamine transmission reflects initiation vigor and exerted effort in an action- and region-specific manner', *Journal of Neuroscience*, 36(7): 2202–11.

Lamm, N. (1974) 'Judaism and the modern attitude to homosexuality', in *Encyclopedia Judaica Year Book*, Jerusalem: Encyclopedia Judaica, pp 194–205.

Lytle, M.C., Blosnich, J.R., De Luca, S.M. and Brownson, C. (2018) 'Association of religiosity with sexual minority suicide ideation and attempt', *American Journal of Preventive Medicine*, 54(5): 644–51.

Momen, M., Bhuiya, A. and Chowdhury, M. (1995) *Vulnerable of the Vulnerables: The Situation of Divorced, Abandoned and Widowed Women in a Rural Area of Bangladesh*, Dhaka, Bangladesh: BRAC-ICDDR,B Joint Research Project, Available from: https://bigd.bracu.ac.bd/wp-content/uploads/2021/11/Vulnerable-of-the-vulnerables-The-situation-of-divorced-abandoned-and-widowed-women-in-a-rural-Area-of-Bangladesh_Working_Paper_11.pdf

National AIDS/STD Programme (2016) '4th National Strategic Plan for HIV and AIDS Response 2018–2022', *UNICEF* [online], Available from: https://www.unicef.org/bangladesh/sites/unicef.org.bangladesh/files/2018-10/NSP%204th%20%202018-2022_draft-250517-2.pdf

Ng, C.H., Guan, M.S., Koh, C., Ouyang, X., Yu, F., Tan, E.K., O'Neill, S.P., Zhang, X., Chung, J. and Lim, K.L. (2012) 'AMP kinase activation mitigates dopaminergic dysfunction and mitochondrial abnormalities in *Drosophila* models of Parkinson's disease', *Journal of Neuroscience*, 32(41): 14311–17.

Olguín, H.J., Guzmán, D.C., García, E.H. and Mejía, G.B. (2016) 'The role of dopamine and its dysfunction as a consequence of oxidative stress', *Oxidative Medicine and Cellular Longevity*, 2016: 9730467. doi: 10.1155/2016/9730467

Paul, A. (2019) 'Geographies of HIV/AIDS in Bangladesh: global perspectives, local contexts and research gaps', in S.T. Islam and A. Paul (eds) *Geography in Bangladesh: Concepts Methods and Applications*, Abingdon: Routledge, pp 54–73.

Raynor, J. (2005) 'Educating girls in Bangladesh: watering a neighbour's tree', in S. Aikman and E. Unterhalterm (eds) *Beyond Access: Transforming Policy and Practice for Gender Equality in Education*, Oxford: Oxfam Publishing, pp 83–105.

Reddy, A., Hoque, M.M. and Kelly, R. (2008) 'HIV transmission in Bangladesh: an analysis of IDU programme coverage', *International Journal of Drug Policy*, 19(Supp 1): 37–46.

Riaz, A. and Rahman, M.S. (eds) (2016) *Routledge Handbook of Contemporary Bangladesh*, Abingdon: Routledge.

Sanzum, T. (2017) 'A deliberate attempt to silence the LGBT community in Bangladesh', *HuffPost* [online], 19 May, Available from: https://www.huffingtonpost.com/entry/a-deliberate-attempt-to-silence-the-lgbt-community-in-bangladesh_us_591f6b5ee4b094cdba542a3f

Stoler, A.L. (1989) 'Rethinking colonial categories: European communities and the boundaries of rule', *Comparative Studies in Society and History*, 31(1): 134–61.

Trading Economics (2021) 'Bangladesh average monthly income' [online], Available from: https://tradingeconomics.com/bangladesh/wages

Tusher, H.J. (2011) 'Rights are equal', *The Daily Star* [online], 8 March, Available from: https://www.thedailystar.net/news-detail-176864

UNICEF (nd) 'Towards ending AIDS: working to secure the goal by 2030' [online], Available from: https://www.unicef.org/bangladesh/en/towards-ending-aids

Urmi, A.Z., Leung, D.T., Wilkinson, V., Miah, M.A.A., Rahman, M. and Azim, T. (2015) 'Profile of an HIV testing and counseling unit in Bangladesh: majority of new diagnoses among returning migrant workers and spouses', *PLOS One* [online], 10(10): e0141483.

Williams, M.E. and Fredriksen-Goldsen, K.I. (2014) 'Same-sex partnerships and the health of older adults', *Journal of Community Psychology*, 42(5): 558–70.

10

Sanjeevani: early ageing and HIV survival in queer Mumbai

Casey Charles

Age is just a number

The AIDS pandemic, now over four decades long, presents complex challenges to our understanding of the process of ageing. The disease itself surely existed before its accepted inception in 1981, and it will continue to plague populations well beyond another 40 years. AIDS has a recorded worldwide death toll of approximately 32 million and currently ranks as one of the longest-lasting plagues, after smallpox (1877–1977; Public Health Online, 2021). Metaphorically, as well, the pandemic has 'grown up' through our understanding of its biological intricacy and our ability to limit its lethal capacity through a series of antiretroviral treatments (ARTs) that have turned what in the 1980s brought an early frost to young men who contracted it into a *chronic* condition that keeps opportunistic infections at bay through protease, integrase and transcriptase inhibitors (Weiss, 2003).

'You are in the middle of your life and you may be at the end of your life at the same time', the Jungian Robert Bosnak remarked to his AIDS patient in his account of their therapeutic journey (1989, p 47). In many ways, the ageing of the pandemic captures the sense of this paradox, but what a pharmacological success story overlooks or, more pessimistically instantiates, is the *nature* of the life that has emerged for HIV long-term survivors (HIVLTS). Without a cure or vaccine, but with a daily drug regimen and its side effects, 21st-century AIDS has created a generation of HIV survivors who, I argue, suffer from early-onset ageing – physically, socially, even psychologically. Certainly, the switch from death sentence to one-pill-a-day undetectability (Olson and Goldstein, 2020) has for certain HIV populations meant a kind of resurrection, but the trauma of diagnosis and the temporary staving off of conditions like herpes, hepatitis and tuberculosis has taken its toll on the best of souls, many of whom must cope with continuing chronic medical conditions. Cardiovascular, osteopathic, neurocognitive, metabolic – such are the kinds of physical comorbidities that face the long-term survivor, whether she is 28 or 68. Immunosenescence in HIVLTS has become a field of medical research (Meir-Shafrir and Pollack, 2012; Tsoukas, 2014). Survivors not only encounter chronic illness but also face the loneliness, isolation and depression sometimes attributed to ageing, especially for a group that must fight stigmas associated with sexual orientation, infectious disease and, if you will, a de facto later life (Robinson et al, 2008).

Even if we accept a more nuanced approach to a strict chronological measure of HIV gerontology, there remains the problem of what social psychologists call the 'stereotyping' of age, namely the way ageism and its negative associations in many cultures, especially queer ones, become a self-perpetuating mental and societal condition (Levy, 2009). For Levy and others, age is to a large degree socially constructed, and regardless of the attribution of body decline and social irrelevance to age, these stereotypes are arguably distributable through a much broader cohort than the older population. The elements of age, under this scenario, are not wedded to a year count or even, I will ultimately argue, to every HIVLTS; they intersect with various factors, including culture, class, ethnicity, sexual orientation and social support systems. There are undetectable 69-year-old positive persons partying and playing with admirable abandon; there are 30-year-old positives who have shut down their social and sexual lives completely.

The stories of three long-term survivors in Mumbai illustrate the complexities of HIV ageing for one particular queer population – a population that must certainly have a lower life expectancy than the 56 years one study, in 2013, attributed to positive 21-year-olds in the US (Mohammadi-Moein et al, 2013; see also Mozes, 2020). None of these HIVLTS from Mumbai is over 50, but most have survived life-threatening illnesses, suicide attempts, drug side effects and stigmatisation. Their survival is also attributable to a social support network that has provided a mechanism for facing the trauma of early-onset ageing. Sanjeevani, the oldest HIV support group for queer men and women in Mumbai, has served as a lifeline for these Mumbaikars, a place of deep intimacy where the trauma of facing the end of life in what should be the middle of it is shared, understood and outlasted.

By focusing on these three individuals from India, a country where viral load assays are still scarce, where antiretrovirals are only available to patients with serious infections, where even HIV testing is not always easily obtainable, I hope to show how the travails of ageing have, as it were, retroactively visited the lives of these 30- and 40-year-olds in the following arenas: physical and medical conditions; mental and emotional challenges; social stigma; and communal support and intimacy. Though later life has come early for these Mumbaikars, they have proved themselves to be long-term survivors.

Group sex

In many ways, a positive HIV test turns youth to age not solely in terms of a compromised immune system but also because of the sudden undesirability of the viral body. Even in the brave new world of highly active ART and undetectability, Grindr is no country for young men rapidly turned old and 'viral'. As a result of the stigma and dangers for long-term survivors, the act of sex often finds a displacement into alternative channels, into what Michel Foucault, in another context, called the 'apparatus of sexuality' – various 'discourses' from pornography to religion, from social work to protest (cited in Weeks, 1986, p 48).[1]

As counter-intuitive as it may seem to impute any sense of erotism to sitting in a circle with a group of strangers who have come together to talk about helper T cells, the HIV/AIDS support group, so endemic to the social trajectory of the pandemic, in many ways partakes of the same spirals of power and pleasure that Foucault (1978, p 45) identified as the confessional mode of the incitement to discourse around sexuality in the 19th century. How did you get it? Who gave it to you? Did the condom break? These questions, often genuine in empathy, share an element of voyeurism, even prurience, in their 'interest' in the 'truth' about participants' sexuality, the excitement of getting to the bottom of another's story. Though the support group – whether it be in India, Kenya or New York – is hardly equivalent to The Stud in San Francisco or a house party, it nonetheless shares an element of erotic charge in its exchange of intimacies. For many HIVLTS, the regular session with peers in various states of health – in venues as varied as church or town hall or online – has served as an interlude of intense intimacy, an opportunity to hug, cry, share, argue, stonewall, even exchange numbers on the sidewalk before heading home. The HIV support group has become an integral part of the sexual history of AIDS.

In Mumbai, Sanjeevani is the oldest HIV support group in the city, having started in 2003, and many of its members, including the participants in this study, ascribe their long-term survival to the cohesion and collective intimacy of this community-based organisation.

This essay and my research into Sanjeevani also participate in the discursive explosion around AIDS and thus also partake of the 'scientia sexualis' that Foucault (1978) describes. Conducted in 2017, these interviews – recorded, translated and retold – became the focus of my naive 'interest', an emotional and intellectual attraction to other HIVLTS queer men and women. I transmit them here, but not before confessing a certain suspect, if not

---

[1] Book Authority (2021) introduces readers to the amazing output on the pandemic. In addition, I am partial to the following websites: The Body (www.thebody.com/); POZ (www.poz.com/); Avert (www.avert.org/), which is now Be in the Know (www.bein theknow.org); My HIV Team (www.myhivteam.com); and UNAIDS (www.unaids.org/ en). Also see the American Psychological Association's list of scientific journals covering HIV: www.apa.org/pi/aids/resources/research/journals.

Orientalist (Said, 1979), epistemological standpoint as a White professor from the United States recounting stories of men who have sex with men (MSM), transgender women and other queer persons from the postcolonial country of India. What standing, what authority have I to represent these narratives given our ethnic, linguistic, economic and global divide? (Jackson, 2021).[2]

Even though the life of a hijra in the megacity of Mumbai is at some levels ungraspable by a cisgender gay man from Montana, what brings us together, nonetheless, is the common ground of HIV long-term survival – the mutual experience of enduring, persevering and ageing during a pandemic without end in sight. My credibility as a chronicler – my standing – derives and gains its validity from my own status as a HIVLTS in his sixties who has, albeit in a different milieu, suffered many of the traumas common to HIVLTS in both India and America, and who seeks 'to heal [my]self and [my] community through understanding, consensus, equality, mutuality' (Baumlin and Meyer, 2018, p 17).

Hanuman

Mumbai is a megacity, one of the most populous in the world with more than 20 million people, its train stations and roads packed tight at all hours, its public bathrooms popular with its sizable MSM population. Death from AIDS dropped 56 per cent between 2010 and 2017, though 43 per cent of the male sex workers in the city and 18 per cent of MSM who visited clinics for sexually transmitted disease (STDs) reported as HIV-positive (Avert, 2020). An estimated 71 per cent of the HIV population has access to antiretrovirals, though stigma and compliance with drug regimens continue to plague the HIV population (Piña et al, 2018). Despite the Supreme Court's decriminalisation of same-sex practices in a landmark court decision in 2018, discrimination continues to play a role in the lives of HIVLTS across India, including the islands of Mumbai, the capital of the state of Maharashtra (Avert, 2020; Human Rights Watch, 2018).

The Humsafar Trust,[3] founded in 1994 by the first out gay journalist in India, Ashok Row Kavi, began as a group support organisation for LGBTIQ Mumbaikars, but the AIDS pandemic quickly transformed the organisation into a health outreach centre, a legal aid office, a major force in the sexual minority community. Now, almost three decades later, it serves close to 100,000 citizens (Humasafar Trust, 2018). When I arrived at the offices of

---

[2] Judith Butler (1990) argues convincingly that essentialism is itself a social construction that seeks to establish a metaphysics of substance, or foundationalism, outside of the discourse that creates identity. For a more recent discussion and critique of essentialism, see Mikkola (2017).

[3] See https://humsafar.org/

Humsafar in 2017, I was ushered into a windowed conference room and introduced to one of the managers, Arjun, a man in his thirties, dressed in slacks and blue oxford shirt, who would be my guide to the handful of interviews I would conduct over the next two days with members of Sanjeevani.[4] Formed in 2003, Sanjeevani, a community-based organisation registered in 2010, is a sub-organisation of Humsafar that came into being through the efforts of a handful of HIV-positive members. Sanjeevani now serves over 300 people living with HIV, MSM, trans and hijra community members through group support, health and nutrition advice, medical and drug assistance, and targeted interventions that include safe sex education, condom distribution, Hepatitis B and C advice, and advocacy.

The name Sanjeevani derives from a magical herb that cures the nervous system and revives people from imminent death. Hanuman, the famous monkey-faced servant of Lord Rama in the *Ramayana*, legendarily travelled to Dronagiri in the Himalayas to collect the herb to help Rama's brother Lakshmana, who was dying from a wound. Hanuman, famous for strength, heroism and devotional love, unable to find the herb, carried the mountain to Lord Rama. The herb has yet to be discovered, but the group understands its name as signalling the healing properties of support while they survive until a cure is found (Balasubranmanian, 2016).

Interviews

Pranit

Pranit is one of the founders of Sanjeevani and certainly considered to be its foremost guru. Many have survived because Pranit convinced them to join Sanjeevani.

He grew up Hindu in Mumbai, mostly happy in childhood but harassed by his two brothers (each more than ten years older), who were ashamed of his 'fem' ways. They tried to teach him to walk like a man, but early on Pranit began to realise he wanted to fall in love with one. "What am I? What is this I am feeling? Is there anyone else?" These questions raced through Pra's head. He was seven or eight; it was the early 1980s. He became rather

---

[4] This was the first of a series of interviews in 2017 with people living with HIV in Mumbai, India, conducted and recorded, with the written permission of participants. The interviews were in some cases translated from Marathi and Hindi. Arjun, fluent in English and Hindi, became my translator during some interviews, presenting my questions to the interviewees and explaining their answers to me. Madhu J. Mitha, a PhD candidate studying in Mumbai and Montana, later translated the interviews in Marathi and Hindi into English. Many of the interviewees spoke some English as well as Hindi, but their extended answers were often recorded in Marathi. I have, after some consideration of privacy issues, decided to change the names of all participants.

camp and his neighbours and schoolmates took advantage of his feminine qualities – sexually. They teased him about being *baila hain* (effeminate), called him a *gandu* (ass fucker). Only when he was 14 or 15 and observed people at the train station did he figure out that there were other twinks like him.

One of his brothers took Pranit a friend's house and after a while, since the friend took interest, left his little brother there. Though Pra knew he liked men, he didn't know how or why God made him the way he was. Meanwhile, his brother's friend started fooling around and eventually ended up fucking Pra, whose ass was sore for days after. Pranit didn't know better; he liked the guy – someone who paid attention to him – even if it hurt. He had just turned 13. No one else cared. His brothers were embarrassed by him, bossing him around and teasing him. Their friends kept yelling, "Hey, your bro is a homo" (*hain*) – that is, not exactly gay, but performatively gay. Pranit's ways came to be a dark mark on the family.

In 1999 Pranit went to the hospital in Mumbai to get tested after a friend from Humsafar convinced him to do this because they had been barebacking. At that point, Pra didn't even know about HIV; he'd just heard of AIDS. The medical community might have been aware of HIV/AIDS in 1999, but in the queer community there was no information, even though people had been dying in New York and San Francisco since the 1980s. In 1999, the Indian government was just beginning to roll out a national programme.

At hospital, they drew blood, and the doctor gave Pranit the results without any counselling. He decided the test results meant he had AIDS. All he knew was that he was going to die, so he headed up to the rooftop terrace to get it over with, to jump off the roof of the hospital. Thank God the door to the terrace was locked. But Pra was isolated – no one to tell, no one to share his fate with. He had seen only one person with AIDS – at the train station in Vile Parle, a man who had a lesion on his nose, a man everyone claimed had AIDS. Pranit saw his own fate in this man hanging out on the platform – he saw the pariah he was destined to become. He stayed home, shut up in shock for many days.

Pranit had always accepted himself sexually, but he only grew to accept HIV with the help of Sanjeevani. Though he grew up Hindu, he has recently converted to Islam. How does he reconcile being Muslim and being queer? The prophets say anal sex is a sin; but then why, Pra asks, did Allah give him this feeling? This is the question that hounds him. On judgment day, he will respectfully ask Allah: If you don't like this kind of sexuality, why did you put this type of feeling in my heart? Pranit belief is that his sexuality is God's gift, that Allah made him the way he is, but asks why he should be condemned and stigmatised for being fem, gay, pos. His answer is that people are put on earth to accept and struggle.

Humsafar saved Pranit's life. He became one of the founders of Sanjeevani and is the mother/father of many of the members, many of whom got tested at his behest, many of whom came to the group with his help, many of whom he cared for as they approached death, men whose families knew nothing of their status or their sexuality. Families showed up at the deathbeds in hospital – amazed, perplexed, ashamed, astounded by the support of Sanjeevani members.

Though he has disclosed his sexuality to most, he guards disclosure of his positivity, in part because he doesn't want to face condescension. He doesn't want sympathy from anyone, except Sanjeevani. These are his people, his family, his intimates. He counsels all the members. Their rallying cry is "Sanjeevani, it will give me a new life!" Pra has had countless friends who have died of AIDS, many of them hastened to their demise through alcohol, which compromises the immune system and impedes adherence to drug regimens. Pra gave up drinking as part of his conversion to Islam. He has had tuberculosis, but never pneumonia, praise Allah. His CD4 count is now 400; he hopes to go higher. He is feeling fine – to the devil with numbers. For Pra, HIV is in his blood, in his body – but not in his mind.

Sanjeevani, he tells me, works with health, nutrition, yoga and social support to keep people living with HIV in a frame of mind that is not focused on sickness unto death, but on survival. He also promotes and believes in the grace of God, a god who is "running all this whole world and what there is in world". Even now, Pra states, many remain ignorant of how the drugs work. There are hundreds of thousands of people in India who just pop a pill and hope it keeps them alive. They have no idea of the importance of adherence. They know nothing of the side effects, nothing about the importance of nutrition and exercise.

Nowadays Pranit's dark skin holds on to a scruffy beard, and instead of the skinny twink he once was, he carries a few extra pounds, his baby blue shirt lighting up his warm smile and radiance. His disarming, forthright and unexpected manner is infectious. He brings you in with his smile, sitting up when I ask about sexual relations.

Pra has had the same lover for many years – a married man, negative and a total top. He lives in Saudi Arabia. They have been together since the turn of the millennium. He is about to return for a visit. They've been together for 14 years, but his guy has been gone for 2 years and probably has had sex. Pra, a total bottom, has gotten used to condoms. His boyfriend is married with two children; his wife does not know about them. If she found out, there would be trouble.

Even with the repeal of the sodomy law, homosexuality remains a major social taboo – no one talks of it. The traditional family structure demands marriage and reproduction. Even straight men who decide not have children are stigmatised. A woman can get another husband if she does not become pregnant. In India, if a girl acts like a boy, many will root for her, but if a boy acts like a girl, it's taboo—he's a pansy. It's patriarchy, sexism, Pra states. There are many, many homophobic men who just want to fuck a tight ass, who want to get or give a blow job but then turn around and hate gays. And there is no counselling for trans or fem men in India – just ridicule, shame, stigma. Nor is there any protection for fem *bois* in schools, even though Pra has gone back to warn his teachers about what is happening with young boys and HIV.

The health minister in India, in total denial, claims their culture does not include same-sex practice among children. This behaviour comes from the West, the minister maintains – an assertion in direct contradiction to the depiction of same-sex behaviours in the temples of Khajuraho, the tenth-century sculptures in Madhya Pradesh (south-east of Delhi). And what about Shikhandi in the *Mahabharata*, the girl who becomes a boy warrior? Official India refuses to recognise its own homoerotic history, Pranit insists.

The government has been completely derelict in providing any information to the people about HIV/AIDS, even in 2017. There is no government-funded outreach, no GIPA[5] in Mumbai. No involvement of the community in policymaking decisions as recommended by the United Nations. There are no free rapid HIV testing centres yet. Pra is quite exercised about how far behind India is lagging – a country with as much expertise and medical know-how as any in the world.

Sanjeevani, he worries, has trouble reaching younger people, in part because the law prevents members from approaching anyone under 18, even though much MSM activity takes place with younger men. Recently the Outreach Project at Humsafar set up a testing station in Thane, in the lake district north of Mumbai. They organised on the internet a gay birthday party. Pra was arrested for handing out condoms and safe-sex information.

Arjun had to go to jail to bail Pranit out. Five people were arrested for having bags of condoms; many of the others were terrified of being outed by the event. They were interrogated like criminals: Did you have sex with someone? Did you take drugs? When Arjun got there, the police held back. They wanted to strip the men and send pictures. The cops wanted bribes. Now in Thane, they do community outreach only informally. Now Humsafar has lawyers to call when the police arrest its members. They do outreach mostly through Facebook, where 8,000 friends have joined.

---

[5] GIPA refers to the UNAIDS commitment to Greater Involvement of People Living with HIV/AIDS, which seeks to strengthen the participation of people living with HIV in the process of continuing their healthy living. GIPA seeks to empower people living with HIV to allow them to become informed, have influence and make decisions around all the medical, economic and social factors that impact the HIV/AIDS community.

Yagnesh

Yagnesh, born in 1981, grew up in Mumbai a happy, happy boy, playing in the streets. A lovely life it was until he discovered he liked boys and realised he was alone. He lived in fear of being found out, ashamed that women did not turn him on. He spent years walking with his head down, afraid of people finding his soul in his eyes, a cloud of shame hanging over him like dust on a dirt road. He soon accepted his queerness as fate, but has never been proud of it. He still has scars on his cheeks where kids bit him. He had to drop out of eighth grade because of bullying. The kids knew he was *baila* (effeminate), and they teased him, tortured him. Yagnesh remembers the day ten men took him to a rooftop and began to gang rape him. His father chased them off in the middle of it. It was filthy. After that incident in the early 1990s, he tested for HIV and, miraculously, was found to be negative.

Yagnesh was betrothed at 10 – an arranged marriage. He now has two children, one boy and one girl – 13 and 11, in ninth and sixth grades. He lives with them and his wife but refuses the label of bisexuality. He wants to be known as gay – just gay. At 18 he was required to get an HIV test by the hospital when his second child was delivered. Both children are negative. When the positive result came back, Yagnesh told his wife she could leave the marriage, but she wanted to stay, wanted him to be her husband even if he had another life. When his wife converted to Christianity, Yag agreed to start praying and going to church, but he is not a Christian. He is Hindu. When he tested positive, he suddenly had to come out about his sexuality to almost everyone he knew, but because he is from a good family, he did not see the worst of it. To his face, no one denigrated him – only behind his back. Up to this day, though, he refuses to go to weddings, like his sisters' celebrations, because of the backlash. He avoids festival season – no Diwali or Holi or Ganpati – except when his HIV support group, his Sanjeevani family, celebrates.

Mostly Yag likes to suck dick in seedy places where men hang out – train stations usually. He used to give tons of blow jobs in Vashi, Neral, and Panvel – areas near or part of Mumbai – where there is a ton of HIV, so he thinks he may have contracted the virus there. Yag found Humsafar in 1999, when he was 18. At the time, he was living with his parents and his wife and working in their shop. He was deeply angry with himself.

One day he met a friend who offered him beer. After getting drunk, he could not go home, so he got on a bus to Neral in suburban Mumbai. When he got off the bus to pee at Neral station, he found the bathroom full of men touching themselves and each other, even having sex. He asked himself in that shocking moment: "Who am I?" He met Ami Jackar there and they talked, Jackar explaining about the down-low in Bombay, about MSM. He handed Yagnesh a slip of paper with the name and number of

Humsafar. Yag called from his parents' landline when he got home, but he didn't go to the centre in East Santacruz until a year later, and the first time he visited, he ran away scared after he encountered a trans guy who told him to never wear gold to the meetings. Finally, he overcame his fear, took courage and attended the Sanjeevani support group. Before long, he was working in the offices of Humsafar.

His seroconversion is still a major mystery, a source of much sorrow. For a long time after he tested positive, he had dark, dark circles around his eyes and was losing sleep because he had no idea where he got the virus. He kept getting tested again and again. Eventually he came to terms with his status and decided that he needed to die. He was confused; his wife found out he was working for Humsafar, a homosexual organisation. He had to tell his family and the pressure of coming out left him sleepless, depressed – uncertain he wanted to exist any more.

He had to reach out for support. Humsafar was the only place he found it. At home, his family and his friends would not talk to him. He made the decision to work for the non-profit, making Rs 6,000 a month, rather than the Rs 30,000 his friends at home were making, which allowed them to buy their own bungalows.[6] He knew he had to stay with Sanjeevani because of his mental health; he knew Humsafar was his only cure. He had to give up money to maintain his heart and well-being in spite of all the pressure from home, where he faced abuse – physical, mental. They hit him and mocked him. Suicide runs in his family like a herd of buffalo. Two of his brothers ended their own lives – one by hanging, the other poison – though neither was HIV related. Yagnesh has tried three or four times to die.

When he found out he was positive after the test at Humsafar, he went home and ate a photo of Madhuri Dixit, the Bollywood actress, that had lived on his wall for many years. He ripped the picture off the wall, tore it up and stuffed the drama queen in his mouth, chasing his feast down with 15 paracetamol tablets. After waking up alive, he gave himself to Humsafar and Sanjeevani, dedicated his life to the survival and health of gay men.

He acquired his first opportunistic infections in 2003 or 2004, when he was around 27. He started to lose his hair, had dark circles under his eyes, grew tired. Yagnesh was scared. He had tuberculosis, but he did not qualify for ARVs because his T cell count was 300. Not until 2010, after two bouts of tuberculosis, when his T cells dropped to 250, did the doctors finally prescribe the drugs. At that time, the CD4 assay was not subsidised, but Humsafar funded half of it. (Now the CD4 assay is free.) Many of Yag's friends had died of tuberculosis, adding to his panic.

---

[6] In 2017, approximately Rs 60 equalled US$1.

Yag now takes a tuberculosis prophylaxis twice a year in the butt, where he has no fat. He is on 'the cocktail'. His T cells have rebounded to 900. He has also battled syphilis. For a long time, he was taking medicine and drinking at night. Now he drinks less alcohol and much more water. His weight has gone from 45 to 82 kilograms – from very thin to very … 'fat' is not a word he likes to articulate. Now he takes the cocktail along with vitamin supplements. He takes nevirapine, lamivudine and azathioprine. Three pills twice a day.

Yagnesh counts 11 different partners over the years. He was faithful to most of them, but usually his lovers ran away and got married. Some were drunks, so he had to leave them. Some harassed Yagnesh for money. They were all *mast* though, all cool in one way. The eleventh, his current partner, is the fulfilment of his dreams – 15 years younger and smaller in build – a hot guy. They don't live together but are an item, talk on the phone every day. Both live at home, so there is no place to shack up, but they go to the cinema and make out. When the family goes to the village, they can steal a day at home. They have spent seven days alone in the house since meeting – in bed mostly. At the beginning of their dating, his lover was violent, pounding on Yag to stop drinking and smoking, to mend his ways, leave the party and play scene so prevalent in the queer community. He is extremely happy but knows marriage is on the horizon for his boy, knows the influence of family pressure on gay men.

Yagnesh's queer name is Jaan Khan. *Jaan* means 'lift'. It's his handle – the name he uses in gay circles. At one point, he figured out he had grown up, was not disco 20 any more. Sanjeevani helped him be real. He has gotten bigger since he showed up there at 19, a skinny boy, beginning work at a time when guys his age were fooling around at house parties. There are no gay bars in Mumbai, he reminds me. Woodhouse Pub closed, and Yag doesn't go to house parties. He'd rather travel around to unknown areas, to chase straight guys. He likes to go to low-key bars and suck dick. He's made friends on Facebook but he does not frequent online dating sites. They didn't start up until around 2012, and Grindr is full of gay men anyway – gay, gay, gay. Not his thing. Every time he goes on Grindr, he only finds men who want beautiful bodies and faces. They want English speakers on Grindr. They want pics and ten-minute hook-ups. They discriminate – gay men do – based on language and colour. There are many bitches on these sites, superficial and racist.

These days in the 2010s, Yagnesh lives three or four different lives. One at the trust, Humsafar, one at home, one when he goes out. At Humsafar and with his friends, everyone knows he's pos – at home, almost no one. With his friends, no one believes him. They say they will never get it; they don't believe he is pos because he is healthy. He only discloses his status when necessary. Why should people have to know if someone has high blood pressure the minute you meet them, he asks, comparing it to his status.

In his free time Yagnesh watches TV – all day. And then calls his boyfriend. Sometimes he hides from his boyfriend and goes to bars to flirt and win over (*pateo*) guys. He shaves, makes himself beautiful and goes to a cheap bar. He just has body sex; he gives blow jobs, just takes it in the mouth. He doesn't fuck; his boyfriend does the fucking. Oral sex on the down-low is his thing. It is the biggest lie of his life – his cottaging, as the Brits call it – his down-low cruising.

He also hides his drinking from his boyfriend, who would beat him if he found out. He is in an open relationship even if his lover doesn't know it. If his lover ever found out, he would scream and abuse Yag, but then be understanding. He would be jealousy incarnate, shouting, hitting Yag. His lover calls himself straight, calls himself MSM. He refuses the term 'gay', and hits. Yag understands; it is very difficult for men to come out in Indian families.

In 2018, Yagnesh turned 40 – round faced, stocky, dark in complexion, soft-spoken. His eyes shine with nervous containment. His goal in life is to help people deal with HIV in a positive way. He wants a cure not just a vaccine. He wants to live his life as fated – as it is written. He wants to teach others to survive, to guide them as they grow older. Each day he takes the medicine, he scolds himself; he feels regret. The medicine confronts him with his disease, but it is written – his fate – and he will live it.

Sanjay

Sanjay was born in Santacruz, a northern suburb in Mumbai, where Humsafar has its office. She was brought up in Vile Parle, a western suburb of Mumbai, known for biscuits, education and the domestic airline Kingfisher. Sanjay was two months old when her mom passed away during a tuberculosis epidemic. Her father remarried and left Sanjay with her beloved grandmother, who raised and supported her as she grew up in the 1980s. Sanjay could not have survived without her.

Her grandma was a housecleaner; sometimes Sanjay went with her to the houses she scrubbed. They lived in a small hut and often went two or three days without food. Grandma would bring home leftovers from the homes she cleaned, and Sanjay would often be home waiting – hungry. She was a studious child, but only stayed in school until the fifth grade. She had to become responsible for her own life before she even knew what the word 'responsibility' meant.

Sanjay doesn't know when she seroconverted, because at the time she was growing up, she didn't know anything about sex or gender. There was no education, and no one spoke about sex in her family or community. It was – and is – taboo. If you are a boy in India, you cannot go out of the house after you are ten years old; you go out only with your family; you go home after work or your family goes after you. Child marriage, technically illegal, is practised through early betrothals, but Sanjay she lived with her grandmother, and lived on almost nothing, there was less pressure on her.

It wasn't until she started working for an insurance company in 1999, at the age of 19, that Sanjay even knew how to travel by train, discover Borivali, Churchgate and Bandra, parts of old Mumbai where they play cricket, parts near the coast where the famous colonial buildings and the Taj Hotel are located. She discovered Andheri, the airport district. The world of Mumbai and the world of her life began to unfold when she got the job. She began wearing platforms to work.

At one of the spots where Sanjay first started to hang out after work, looking for sex, Humsafar workers would come around and hand out condoms. Before that, she knew nothing of safe sex. She first met her hijra mom, Pranit, there. It was Pranit who convinced Sanjay to get tested. When she found out she was positive, Sanjay felt blank; she had to ask Pra what the test meant. Pranit told her she was not going to die, but it took Sanjay time to accept that. Pranit told her there were many, many living with HIV; but for many at that time HIV meant AIDS and AIDS meant death – pure and simple. Who would take care of her grandmother if she died?

Poverty took Sanjay's childhood away; HIV stole her twenties from her. She had to worry about safer sex and transmission, and though not as dire as starving, living with the virus impeded her life and gave her many, many hours of tears. She never told her grandmother she was positive even though Grandma knew most everything about her. She even met Sanjay's first boyfriend, who was also an outreach worker. He slept over a couple of times at their house. She also supported Sanjay during her decision to transition from male to female, which began when she was 25 (Chakrapani, 2010).[7] Her grandma helped her to get ready for drag shows, since back then there was no green room and she had to dress and do her make-up before leaving home in a sari or sharara for the Lavani dances. Her neighbours soon discovered she was hijra, but they supported her, even hired an autorickshaw to take her to her events so she would not be harassed on the street.[8] Sanjay doesn't live in Parle any more but goes back to the district where her grandma lived, to visit her amazing neighbours.

---

[7] Sanjay is a hijra, but also identifies as transgender. Chakrapani (2010) discusses the discrete connections and disconnections between the historical hijra culture and the current transgender designation.

[8] Hijra broadly refers to a person whose gender is neither male nor female, typically a person born male who dresses as a woman. In India, hijra can also refer to a transgender or transitioning person. India's Supreme Court has recognised hijra as a third gender (Khaleeli, 2014).

When her grandmother died, Sanjay directed all the arrangements. She was planning the funeral at a time when she had begun hormone therapy – her breasts improving somewhat, her hair very, very long. Her father refused to do the final rites, but Sanjay shaved her head in keeping with Hindu practice to cut off part of one's body to give to the gods. Sanjay shaved her head even though this is primarily a male practice – out of respect for her grandma.

After testing positive in 1999, she interviewed with Humsafar and became an MSM outreach worker. She learned to deal with the tensions and phobias among MSM, trans and gay communities. Transgenders can face a triple stigma: as queer, as gender outlaws and often as sex workers (Chakrapani et al, 2017; Ganju and Saggurti, 2017). And most hijras are very poor and live in the slums. Sanjay's job involves distribution of condoms and information about STDs. She is often not welcome; hijra houses tell her to leave the condoms and get out. HIV stigma looms on top of these other stigmas. If you test positive, whether you are guru or chela, you are typically kicked out of your house.[9] The guru almost invariably buys a bus ticket for the chela and sends her back to her village. No one, Sanjay insists, wants to get infected by a pos chela.

Hijra culture is very hierarchical. *Gurua-sishya-parampara* (a teacher student relationship – guru/chela, mother/daughter) exists as a traditional form of sociality. Hijras live by dancing (*Nach Gaana*), singing, going to marriages, blessings, sex work, begging – dressed in sparkling saris and wearing gobs of make-up. Over the years, Sanjay herself has adopted four chelas, though only two of them know about her HIV status. They are in different *gharanas* or households. She never discloses her status when she stands on the roadside for clients, because if her clients knew, she would get no business. She just practises safe sex. More often than not, Sanjay has watched pos hijras become depressed, lose work, start drinking. Sanjay tries to avoid depression by going inside herself, removing herself from the scene for a while. She currently has a boyfriend but she fears losing him to marriage.

Sanjay is 44 now; she grew up with Humsafar, and Humsafar, now a national non-governmental organisation, grew up with her. She is now a community counsellor, the trans point person who is prominently in the news. She travelled to the United States for a trans health symposium and last year was invited to a South African conference, which published one of her papers.

The percentage of HIV positivity in the trans community is even higher than in the gay community in India – almost 20 per cent by some accounts. 'High fun' has become a trend in the MSM and trans world in India. This

---

[9] Guru is teacher and chela, disciple. In hijra social structure, every chela has a mother or guru who protects and fosters her disciples (Countries and their Cultures, 2021).

involves party and play and often group sex, risky popper-taking gang sex. Add the ingredient of alcohol and the risk of sexual transmission becomes major. Many sex workers, including Sanjay when she was super active, have 10–15 clients in one night. Often cheaters come with clients; police come. All want to fuck. Alcohol is the only means of alleviating the stress. Many trans sisters have passed away, not just from AIDS but also Hepatitis B.

After resisting the cocktail for many years, Sanjay's CD4 fell to 212. The doctors convinced her to take the drugs. Regaining her health, she adopted the role of helping her trans sisters, and now it has taken over her life. Sanjay has morphed into an activist and social worker.

Shakti, Shakti

Sanjeevani's philosophy of hope drives the group's belief in a cure – medical as well as social. Shakti is cosmic experience and liberation; it is a psychospiritual force that inspires everyone at the end of meetings to hold hands and sing the 16th-century hymn (Tulsidas, 2013):

> *Shakti Hame Dena*
> *Itni shakti hume dena data*
> *Man ka vishwas kamzor ho no*
> *Hum chalen nek raste pe hamse*
> *Bhoolkar bhi koi bhool ho na*

> [Give us so much strength, O Lord,
> that the faith of our heart never waivers.
> May we walk the path of goodness
> and make no mistake even accidentally.
> Give us so much, O Lord
> that the faith in our hearts never waivers]

For the members of Sanjeevani, many of whom had faced a lifetime of travails by the time they reached 30, these lyrics and the memory of held hands becomes a mantra for survival and support they carry with them from meeting to meeting.

Examining the lives of queer HIVLTS in Mumbai highlights the way the challenges of ageing are not determined by a numerical threshold. A life-threatening illness like HIV not only hastens the ageing process but also forces individuals into an existential crisis, a moment of truth which demands either resistance and survival or succumbing to sickness. In the queer community of Mumbai, where life span, stigma, family pressure and medical scarcity continue to create serious adversities, these men and women in their thirties and forties have already overcome a lifetime of obstacles, attesting to the way the experience of later life, with or without HIV, is a struggle for survival and resistance, during which new forms of intimacy can unfold. Sanjeevani has created the foundation for perseverance and even pleasure. The result is tenacity and tenderness through togetherness as we wait for a cure.

References

Avert (2020) 'At a glance: HIV in India' [online], Available from: https://www.avert.org/professionals/hiv-around-world/asia-pacific/india

Balasubranmanian, D. (2016) 'In search of the Sanjeevani plant of Ramayana', *The Hindu* [online], 17 December, Available from: https://www.thehindu.com/sci-tech/science/In-search-of-the-Sanjeevani-plant-of-Ramayana/article16880681.ece

Baumlin, J.S. and Meyer, C.A. (2018) 'Positioning ethos in/for the twenty-first century: an introduction to histories of ethos', *Humanities* [online], 7(3): 78, Available from: http://dx.doi.org/10.3390/h7030078

Book Authority (2021) '77 best HIV books of all time' [online], Available from: https://bookauthority.org/books/best-hiv-books

Bosnak, R. (1989) *Dreaming with an AIDS Patient*, Boston, MA: Shambhala.

Butler, J. (1990) *Gender Trouble: Feminism and the Subversion of Identity*, New York: Routledge.

Chakrapani, V. (2010) *Hijras/Transgender Women in India: HIV, Human Rights and Social Exclusion*, Issue Brief, United Nations Development Programme, India, Available from: https://archive.nyu.edu/bitstream/2451/33612/2/hijras_transgender_in_india.pdf

Chakrapani, V., Newman, P.A., Shunmugam, M., Logie, C.H. and Samuel, M. (2017) 'Syndemics of depression, alcohol use, and victimization, and their association with HIV-related sexual risk among men who have sex with men and transgender women in India', *Global Public Health*, 12(2): 250–65.

Countries and their Cultures (2021) 'Hijra – kinship and social organization' [online], Available from: https://www.everyculture.com/South-Asia/Hijra-Kinship-and-Social-Organization.html

Foucault, M. (1978) *The History of Sexuality, Volume 1: An Introduction*, trans R. Hurley, New York: Pantheon.

Ganju, D. and Saggurti, N. (2017) 'Stigma, violence and HIV vulnerability among transgender persons in sex work in Maharashtra, India', *Culture, Health & Sexuality*, (19)8: 903–17.

Human Rights Watch (2018) 'India: Supreme Court Strikes Down Sodomy Law' [online], 6 September, Available from: https://www.hrw.org/news/2018/09/06/india-supreme-court-strikes-down-sodomy-law#

Humsafar Trust (2018) [online] Available from: https://humsafar.org/

Jackson, J.B. (2021) 'On cultural appropriation', *Journal of Folklore Research*, (58)1: 77–122.

Khaleeli, H. (2014) 'Hijra: India's third gender claims its place in law', *The Guardian* [online], 16 April, Available from: https://www.theguardian.com/society/2014/apr/16/india-third-gender-claims-place-in-law

Levy, B. (2009) 'Stereotype embodiment: a psychosocial approach to aging', *Current Directions of Psychological Science*, (18)6, 332–336.

Meir-Shafrir, K. and Pollack, S. (2012) 'Accelerated aging in HIV patients', *Ramban Maimonides Medical Journal*, 3(4): e0025. doi:10.5041/RMMJ.10089

Mikkola, M. (2017) 'Gender essentialism and anti-essentialism', in A. Garry, S.J. Khader and A. Stone (eds) *The Routledge Companion to Feminist Philosophy*, New York: Routledge, pp 168–76.

Mohammadi-Moein, H.R., Maracy, M.R. and Tayeri, K. (2013) 'Life expectancy after HIV diagnosis based on data from the Counseling Center for Behavioral Diseases', *Journal of Research in Medical Sciences: The Official Journal of Isfahan University of Medical Sciences*, 18(12), 1040–5.

Mozes, A. (2020) 'Despite medical advances, people with HIV still live shorter, sicker lives', *Medical Press* [online], Available from: https://medicalxpress.com/news/2020-06-medical-advances-people-hiv-shorter.html

Olson, R.M. and Goldstein, R. (2020) 'U=U: ending stigma and empowering people living with HIV', *Harvard Health Publishing* [online], Available from: https://www.health.harvard.edu/blog/uu-ending-stigma-and-empowering-people-living-with-hiv-2020042219583

Piña, C., Dange, A., Rawat, S., Jadhav, U., Arnsten, J.H., Chhabra, R. and Patel, V.V. (2018) 'Antiretroviral treatment uptake and adherence among men who have sex with men and transgender women with HIV in Mumbai, India: a cross-sectional study', *Journal of the Association of Nurses in AIDS Care*, 29(2): 3210–16.

Public Health Online (2021) 'The worst global pandemics' [online], Available from: https://www.publichealthonline.org/worst-global-pandemics-in-history/

Robinson, W.A., Petty, M.S., Patton, C. and Kang, H. (2008) 'Aging with HIV: historical and intra-community differences in experience of aging with HIV', *Journal of Gay and Lesbian Social Services*, 201(1–2), 111–28.

Said, E.W. (1979) *Orientalism*, New York: Vintage.

Tsoukas, C. (2014) 'Immunosenescence and aging in HIV', *Current Opinion in HIV and AIDS*, 9(4): 398–404.

Tulsidas (2013) *Hanuman Chalisa*, Gorakhpur, India: Gita Press, Available from: https://web.archive.org/web/20121119071944/http://www.gitapress.org/books/1528/1528%20Hanuman%20chalisa.pdf

Weeks, J. (1986) *Sexuality*, New York: Tavistock Publications.

Weiss, R.A. (2003) 'HIV and AIDS in relation to other pandemics', *EMBO Reports*, (Suppl 1): S10–S14.

Afterword

Mark Henrickson

HIV is not over.

Venerable (how they would hate that word!) AIDS organisations such as Gay Men's Health Crisis (GMHC) in New York and the AIDS Action Committee of Boston began reminding us as long ago as 1989 that despite astonishing advances in treatments, HIV is not over. I have a faded refrigerator magnet from GMHC that reminds me of those words every day. The World Health Organization (2021) continues to remind the world that HIV and HIV stigma are ongoing global realities.

The lives of people living with HIV are not over. This is equally important to remember.

The contributors to this book have shared stories of people from all over the world who are living with HIV in what they consider later life (however old in years they may be), people still coping with the stigmas associated with both HIV and with later life. Antiretroviral treatments have worked their medical magic in places where they are readily accessible, and people with HIV are living their lives with less physical suffering, with less risk of early death. People with HIV are no longer 'standing in the fire', as one African research participant told me years ago (Fouché et al, 2011). That is an astonishing and wonderful thing. But the stories we have heard in this volume are not only, or even mostly, about people living with HIV; they are also about people living with the stigma associated with HIV, as though their lives *should* be over. Women in Switzerland, Ukraine and the United Kingdom who have withdrawn from their communities and who avoid emotional and sexual relationships; gay men in the United Kingdom and Aotearoa New Zealand who continue to marginalise older gay men; gay men, women, trans women and hijra living with HIV; Kenyans and South Asians living with HIV and marginalised identities – these and others who no longer need others to stigmatise them, because they have learned so well to stigmatise themselves. People living with HIV find support in other people living with HIV, and they have drawn together to protect each other against the stigma and malice of a stigmatising world. It is only the few courageous voices who risk telling their stories. To those who have shared their personal stories in this book, and for research participants who have shared their stories with researchers, we are grateful.

The title of this book, *HIV, Sex and Sexuality in Later Life*, risks misdirecting the gaze of the reader. In understanding more about the experiences of people in later life living with HIV, the critical gaze of caregivers, policymakers and researchers must be focused not on people living with HIV, but rather on people, policies and providers who stigmatise and marginalise. That is a central theme of all these stories from every part of the world. Those of us who live with or work in HIV/AIDS learned early on that we should not use the word 'victims' (as in 'AIDS victims'). The notion of victim is disempowering and implies that HIV robs people of their agency, their ability to advocate for and to look after themselves. From the beginning of the epidemic, people living with HIV and those who love them reminded caregivers and policymakers that they had plenty of power. It would not be an overstatement to say that HIV transformed the way medical care is delivered throughout the world. No longer are 'patients' passive recipients of medical wisdom, following directions and doing as they are told by unassailably wise providers. Drug trials, drug approval processes, care providers, researchers and policymakers responded to activist pressure to expedite new treatments, to be more inclusive, to understand the person as an active participant in treatment decisions. They began to understand that HIV was as much a social diagnosis as a medical one. HIV activists who refused to be victims transformed healthcare around the world.

Yet the same cannot be said about stigma. 'People living with stigma' is not quite accurate, not quite complete, because although people living with HIV certainly live with stigma, stigma is a socially created and agreed reality, like sexism, homophobia, racism and the other isms of privilege. Of course we can educate to try to prevent stigma, we can protest stigma, we can have all manner of public campaigns to address stigma, as we do other isms, but still, as we have seen in these chapters, stigma about HIV remains intractable. AIDS organisations around the world maintain the elimination of stigma and discrimination as a goal (Henrickson et al, 2017), as do global AIDS organisations (see UNAIDS, 2021). Yet stigma remains stubbornly prevalent, unresponsive to treatment; humans seem to need to create 'others' to assure themselves at least of who they are not. We apparently need the intersectional isms in order to maintain our privileges and power. To relegate people living with HIV in later life to a top shelf in a cupboard so that they are out of sight is to try to control them, to avoid what may be messy and complex lives, reminders of the failures of our social and healthcare systems. A goal of this volume is to encourage caregivers and policymakers not to participate in that stigma by assuming that the emotional, sexual and relational lives of people living with HIV in later life – and more and more people living with HIV are in the latter part of their lives – are over. They are not. The assumption that older people should 'behave', that they are not attractive, that people living with HIV in later life are somehow not deserving of love and relationships – these merely reproduce ageist and cis-heteronormative assumptions and privileged discourses about how people 'should' live their lives. Part of what living with HIV has done in the era of highly active antiretroviral therapy and pre-exposure prophylaxis is to allow and encourage people to reclaim all of their lives, and those lives include sex and sexuality, free from the judgements and assumptions of otherness.

Not a few people have noticed the parallels between HIV and the most recent global pandemic of COVID-19 (Rickard, 2021). The world's willingness to marginalise and stigmatise vulnerable groups has a regrettably long history, quite probably stretching back to prehistory. It would be reassuring to be able to say that despite the devastation brought about by HIV at the end of the 20th century, the world learned something from our experience, but it seems we have not. Although we will hear most about its medical, social and economic effects on the rich world, inevitably COVID-19, like HIV, will affect the poorest, most marginalised, most vulnerabilised communities of people around the world. As will the next pandemic, and the one after that, and climate change, and all the many apocalyptic ills of our planet. *HIV, Sex and Sexuality in Later Life* is not merely about HIV, sex and sexuality in later life: it is about challenging the assumptions, expectations and privileges that each of us carries; about how to be competent caregivers and policymakers; and ultimately about how to be good global citizens.

References

Fouché, C., Henrickson, M., Poindexter, C., Scott, K., Brown, D.B. and Horsford, C. (2011) *"Standing in the Fire": Experiences of HIV-Positive Black African Migrants and Refugees Living in New Zealand*, Auckland, Aotearoa New Zealand: University of Auckland, Available from: http://community research.org.nz/research/standing-in-the-fire-experiences-of-hiv-posit ive-black-african-migrants-and-refugees-living-in-new-zealand/

Henrickson, M., Chipanta, D., Lynch, V.J., Muñoz Sanchez, H., Nadkarni, V.V., Semigina, T. and Sewpaul, V. (eds) (2017) *Getting to Zero: Global Social Work Responds to HIV*, Geneva, Switzerland: IASSW and UNAIDS, Available from: http://www.unaids.org/en/resources/documents/2017/ global-social-work-responds-to-HIV

Rickard, S. (2021) 'Doctor describes HIV/AIDS epidemic and COVID-19 pandemic parallels as "hauntingly similar"', *Spectrum News 1* [online], Available from: https://spectrumlocalnews.com/tx/south-texas-el-paso/ news/2021/07/09/doctor-describes-hiv-epidemic--covid-19-pandemic-as--hauntingly-similar-

UNAIDS (2021) 'Stigma and discrimination' [online], Available from: https:// www.unaids.org/en/keywords/stigma-and-discrimination

World Health Organization (2021) 'Why the HIV epidemic is not over' [online], Available from: https://www.who.int/news-room/spotlight/ why-the-hiv-epidemic-is-not-over

Index

References to endnotes show both the
page number and the note number (231n3).